CREATIVE FACE

make your own makeup

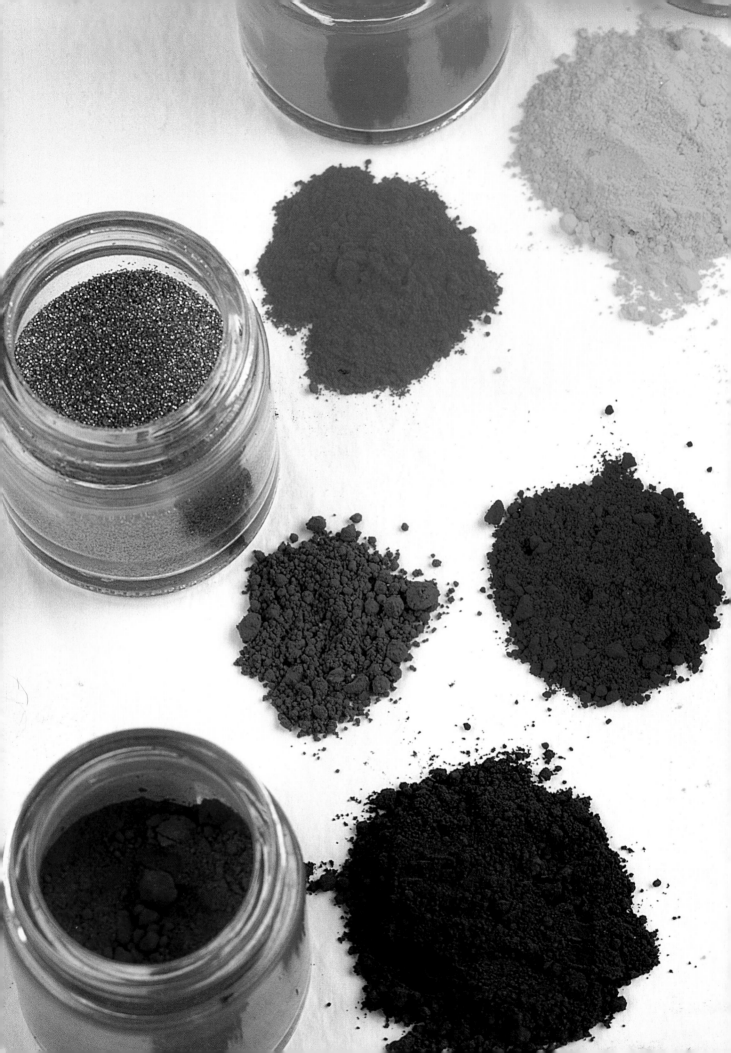

CREATIVE FACE

make your own makeup

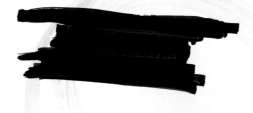

maxine nelson

sixth&spring books

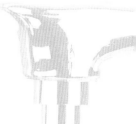

First published in 2005 in the USA by

Sixth&Spring Books
An Imprint of Soho Publishing Company
233 Spring St, 8th floor
New York, NY 10013

First published in 2004 in the UK
By New Holland Publishers
Garfield House
86-88 Edgware Rd
London W2 2EA

Library of Congress Control Number: 2004109339

ISBN: 1-931543-62-3

Senior Editor: Clare Hubbard

Photographer: Shona Wood

Design: Bridgewater Book Company

Production: Hazel Kirkman

Editorial Direction: Rosemary Wilkinson

Cover design: Chi Ling Moy

Manufactured in Malaysia

1 3 5 7 9 10 8 6 4 2

Disclaimer
The author and publishers have made every effort to ensure that all instructions, storage, sterilization and application methods given in this book are safe and accurate, but they cannot accept liability for any resulting injury or loss or damage to either property or person, whether direct or consequential and howsoever arising.

The makeup made using the recipes in this book is for personal use only, it cannot be sold.

The advice on color additives has been carefully documented from various sources. The D.T.I, the E.U., Warner Jenkins (Europe), Kingfisher Colours (UK) and the F.D.A. have all supplied information deemed as correct at the time of going to press. Subdivisions of regulations occur in certain countries. If a product is deemed unsuitable in your home country, please substitute it with a shade variation. Your supplier will be able to find an alternative.

All of the recipes are suitable for most skin types, however due to sensitivities in some individuals, the author and publishers accept no responsibility for misinterpretation or reactions to products which might occur. It is recommended that you test each product that you make on a small area of skin before using it fully.

The publishers have made every effort to ensure that the information contained in this book was correct at the time of going to press.

Acknowledgements
My sincere thanks go to: Rachel Rawicki, whose enthusiasm and eye for color was inspiring; To Darren, my wonderful husband, who supports my boundless ideas and made living in France the most perfect time of my life; Tilly, Bizzy, Gemma (my beautiful daughters), Charlotte Rawicki and my son Stephen's partner lola for being recipe testers and models; Jayne and Remy Gellar NYC for working with me on the ingredient supplies; last but never least, Melinda Coss, whose faith in me made this possible.

CONTENTS

INTRODUCTION

Being able to make cosmetics and toiletries out of natural ingredients inspired me to look at the possibilities of making my own makeup. My interest in makeup started at a very early age. The center of most people's homes is the kitchen; in my home it was my mother's dressing table. My mother Eileen was a model in the late 1950s, early 1960s. I would sit on the corner of her bed listening to stories of beautiful clothes, travels, and modeling assignments. On her French-styled dressing table were a wonderful array of bottles and jars, lipsticks, panstick foundation, and, of course, mascara in cake form with the flat little brush.

The history of makeup goes back many thousands of years to cave dwellers painting their bodies with roots, berries, fats, and clays. Many of the very early makeup recipes contained lead powders, so alternatives were sought. The early chemists found ways of isolating ingredients in natural products and replicating them in a laboratory, therefore making a synthetic from a natural. Now we are discovering that many natural substances need to remain "whole" to be effective.

The idea of using natural materials and ingredients was the beginning of my interest in aromatherapy, perfumery, soaps, and cosmetics. This led to further studies in the science of cosmetics. I felt that it had to be possible to make eye shadows, lipsticks, and many other products using mainly natural ingredients. My first task was to find out how commercial manufacturers made their products. Having discovered some of their methods, I began to wonder whether homemade makeup would be effective? Would it be possible to achieve a neat finish without the use of high-tech machinery? After much experimenting, I discovered that it was.

Natural ingredients do not have the same long-lasting shelf-life of some chemical products, but with careful use and attention to hygiene, they combine to make a perfectly safe product. Makeup often remains in bags and drawers for years, but by making your own fresh makeup, this is a thing of the past. Before you start making your makeup, please read the disclaimer on page 4 and all of the introductory sections (pages 8–19). In these pages you'll find all of the essential information about equipment, ingredients, storage, applicators, and safety.

We abuse our skin by scrubbing it, and shaving it; we pick it, pierce it, expose it to extremes of heat and cold, and squash it into clothes and shoes. It makes sense to limit the amount of chemicals we inflict on it by knowing what goes into our makeup and using natural ingredients wherever possible.

RIGHT *Blusher is just one of the products that you can make at home (see pages 68–69).*

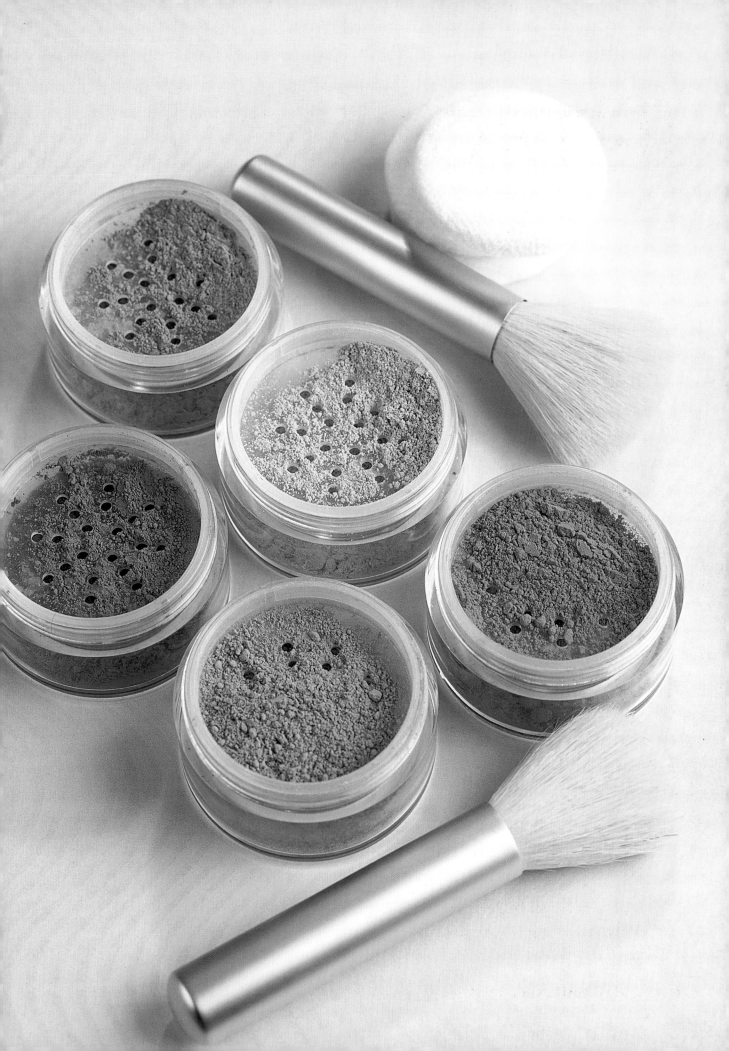

EQUIPMENT

Much of the equipment that you need is standard kitchen equipment, but for hygiene reasons you should buy a new set of everything and use it only for making makeup. You will find most of the products in local stores, or you can contact one of the suppliers listed on page 94.

Aluminum foil and plastic wrap for molding and wrapping sticks and lipsticks.

Assortment of containers and jars in which you will store your finished makeup (see pages 16–17).

Assortment of bowls (glass and plastic) for storing ingredients and heating mixtures. Always make sure that you use the appropriate bowl for the task; i.e when melting fats and waxes, use a heat-resistant bowl.

Coffee stirrers or popsicle sticks for stirring small quantities of mixture.

Coin or counter (die) for pressing on the surface of eye shadows to flatten them.

Dropper or pipette from an old flower-remedy bottle or eye-dropper.

Eggbeater for blending and dispersing ingredients in mixtures.

Icing bag with doughnut, cream, or jam filler nozzle is useful for filling small tubes and jars.

Isopropyl alcohol or similar sterilizing agent for sterilizing equipment and containers. Sterilizing solution used for babies' bottles is ideal.

Juice squeezer for extracting juice from lemons for recipes.

Measuring cups or glass measuring beakers are useful, 10ml–100ml. They should be heat-resistant.

Measuring spoons are essential. It is advisable to use stainless steel ones as they are easier to clean than plastic. I favor a set of ¼ to 1 teaspoon size and a set of "pinch, smidgen and dash" spoons. For teaspoon measures and fractions, use the measurements as a guide. You can halve or double the amount of ingredient depending on how much you wish to make.

Paper towels are generally useful to have around, particularly to protect your work surface when using color powders, as a tiny grain goes a long way.

Pens or pencils to use as a template for sticks and lipsticks (average lipstick diameter is ½ in).

Pestle and mortar for grinding powders and ingredients.

Pointed nozzle bottle for Henna Paste recipe (see page 77).

Potholder or oven glove for holding beakers or pans containing hot liquids/melted wax.

Rubber stamps can be used to make an impression in the surface of compacted eye shadows.

Saucepans should be stainless steel as non-stick pans may peel and contaminate the makeup, and aluminum may react with oils and damage the mixture. A double boiler is essential for melting fats and waxes; otherwise, rest a heat-resistant bowl over a pan of hot water.

Scales need to be very accurate and preferably be able to weigh as little as 1g. It is best if they are the sort that can be returned to "zero" so that you can add multiple ingredients into one container.

Strainer for straining herbal infusions or dispersing powders before mixing. (A fine tea strainer can also be used.)

Syringe for accurately dispensing liquids. A simple medicine dispenser syringe (often used for cough syrup for small children) is ideal.

Thermometer – a lab type is the best, although a glass or steel meat thermometer will be adequate.

Thin latex gloves protect your hands when using products that may stain the skin (i.e. henna).

Tip

In many recipes I refer to using a "matchhead" of an ingredient. This circle ● *represents how much that is — roughly the size of a head of a matchstick.*

BELOW *Most of the equipment required is standard kitchenware, but it is essential to buy new equipment before you start making your own makeup.*

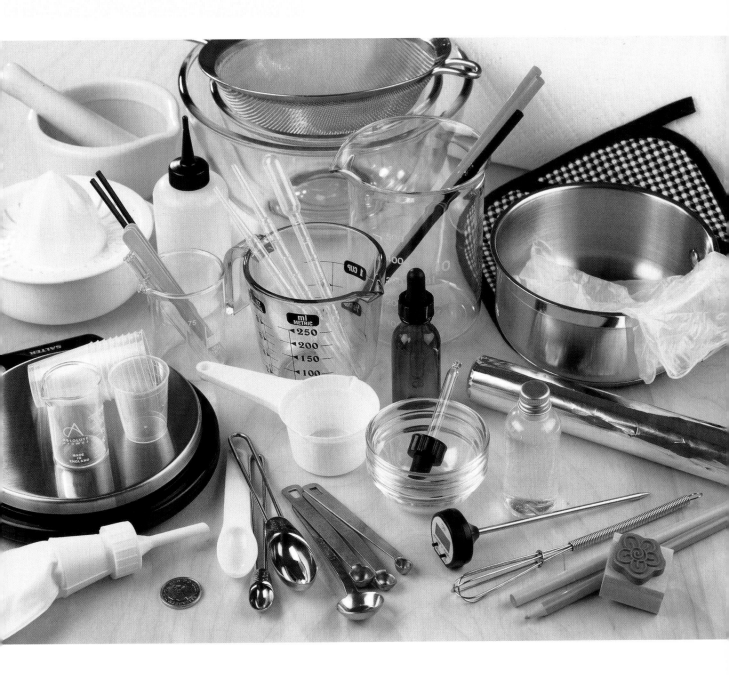

INGREDIENTS

Makeup is a color cosmetic that gently adheres to your skin. It needs several elements to make it effective – covering power, absorbancy, adhesion, staying power, and bloom (matte and silky appearance). Most commercially produced makeup is packed full of preservatives, silicones, and numerous other components that have varying roles to produce effective products. Many are waterproof, runproof, creaseproof, and often have chemical meshes in a microscopic film to make them aesthetically pleasing when the lid is removed. Many products also contain ingredients to protect the container from being damaged by the product. The ingredients in my recipes are mainly of natural vegetable or mineral origin, or gentle additives that work in harmony with the skin. I have tried to use natural products whenever possible, but for stability and safety even natural products sometimes require rectifying to make them suitable for use on the skin. One of the most powerful poisons known to the human race is a natural product taken from castor beans, yet when refined, castor (bean) oil is one of the most important and safe oils to use in lipstick manufacture.

I have kept the recipes as simple as possible in order to produce effective cosmetics while using the minimum number of components. Unless stated otherwise, you cannot substitute ingredients as each has a valuable purpose in the recipe. Most of the ingredients can be obtained in drugstores, craft stores, or health food centers. Check with your suppliers; some sell in quantities as small as 10g or 10ml depending on the cost of the product. Color powders can sometimes be obtained from craft stores but obviously you must make sure that they are suitable for use in cosmetics. The best options for buying cosmetic-quality colorants are the specialized mail-order companies, listed on pages 94–95.

The formulations require a medium (powder, oil, or cream) in which the color is dispersed. The natural powder bases contain cornstarch, natural talcum, magnesium stearate (made from palm oil), potato starch, and powdered colorants. The fats, oils, and waxes include shea butter, cocoa butter, jojoba oil, beeswax, and vitamin E. When a recipe contains water, you must use purified water. Water and oil do not mix freely, so it is necessary to add emulsifiers. An emulsifier will assist in the binding together of the oil and water mixture (emulsion). Beeswax, fatty alcohols, and modified waxes are all emulsifiers.

Many people perceive that natural products lack glamor. This is simply not the case. Makeup with a natural base can be both a professional-quality product and extremely glamorous. The color pigments used can be a selection from nature as it intended – assisted or replicated. Think of sparkling jewels such as sapphires or emeralds, wonderful semiprecious stones, gold, copper, and silver found deep in the earth, and brightly colored flower petals.

Apple cider vinegar Restores the skin's natural pH levels, provided it is diluted first as directed in the recipe.

Almond oil (*Prunus dulcis*) Sweet almond oil is used as an emollient, for massage, and in ointments and creams.

Aloe vera (*Aloe barbadensis*) Soothing and protective, one of the oldest medicinal healing plants. Naturally oxygenates the skin and is good for cell renewal.

Apricot kernel oil (*Prunus armeniaca*) Similar to sweet almond oil, but is lighter on the skin. Has a high vitamin E content. Helps the skin retain elasticity.

Aromaflavors Water- or glycerin-based food-grade products suitable for flavoring lip cosmetics.

Benzoin resinoid Healing, soothing, and has some preservative qualities. May help heal broken and cracked skin. Resin is diluted to become a pourable liquid.

Beeswax (cosmetic) (*Cera alba*) Used in a variety of recipes as an emulsifier. May have healing and antiseptic properties. Stiffens wax- and oil-blended products.

Calendula macerated oil Anti-inflammatory; amazing healing powers on the skin and scar tissue. Flowers are soaked (macerated), usually in a sunflower or olive oil base, then the oil is strained for use.

Carnauba wax (*Copernicia cerifera*) A "wax" that is solid at room temperature. Also known as Brazilian Palm Wax. A barrier, lubricating and texturizing.

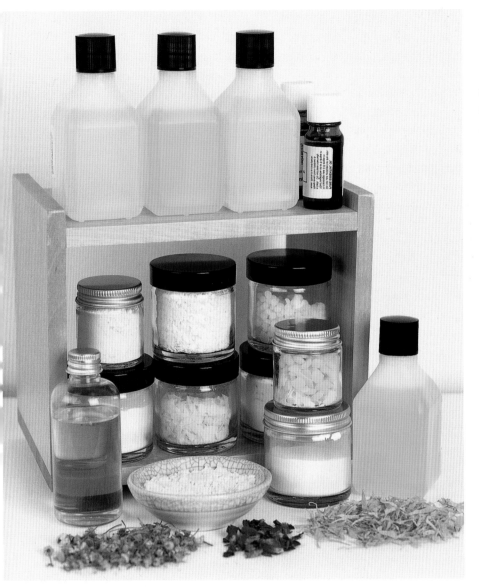

Carrot oil Packed with vitamin A, good for skin regeneration.

Castor oil (*Ricinus communis*) A barrier oil with emollient and lubricating properties.

Cedarwood essential oil (*Cedrus atlantica*) Helps clear oil-rich skin of a buildup of sebum and has healing qualities.

Cetyl alcohol This is not a liquid, but comes in the form of white flakes. Used for its emollient and emulsifying properties. Close resemblance to certain constituents of sebum.

Clary sage essential oil (*Salvia sclaria*) Healing and balancing, particularly for combination skin. Works well with anti-inflammatory preparations.

Cocoa butter (*Theobroma cocoa*) Hard fat (butter) with emollient and mild sunscreen properties.

Cornstarch (*Zea mays*) White powdered corn, which is mild on the skin and widely used in skin-care products and makeup.

Emulsifying wax Product that prevents oil and water from separating in creams and lotions. May be of alcohol and/or vegetable origin.

Evening primrose oil (*Oenothera biennis*) High linoleic acid (G.L.A) content. Rehydrates and revitalizes the skin. Soothes and calms inflammation and increases the skin's elasticity.

Frankincense (*Boswellia carterii*) Particularly beneficial for mature and devitalized skin.

Geranium essential oil (*Pelargonium graveolens*) Good for balancing combination skin; keeps harmony when the skin and mind feel off-balance.

Germaben II A preservative.

Glycerin Water-attracting, binding ingredient produced during soap manufacture. Can be of animal or vegetable (soap) origin, but I have used only the vegetable origin product in my recipes.

Guar gum Thickener and emulsifier originating from the *Cyamopsis tetragonoloba* plant. A complex carbohydrate.

Honey A natural emollient, with healing, hydrating, and antiseptic properties.

Hydrolats/hydrosols/floral waters Water solution containing energizing properties or constituents made by distilling plant material or petals. In the distillation of essential oils, the pure essential oil naturally separates, and the remaining condensed water has strong therapeutic and fragrant properties.

Jojoba oil (*Simmondsia chinensis*) A "wax" that is molten at room temperature. Very light texture on the skin and is said to be similar to human sebum. Moisturizing and good for cell renewal.

Kaolin (China clay) Good for absorbing oil from the skin. Gives slip to powder makeup.

Lavender essential oil (*Lavandula angustifolia*) The best known and most widely used healing, soothing, relaxing, and balancing oil. Helps reduce scarring and stimulates the growth of healthy skin cells.

Lemon juice Natural lemon juice acts as a mild preservative, antioxidant, and pH balancer.

Lecithin A natural antioxidant and emollient; also makes a product easier to apply and spread.

Magnesium stearate Natural "soap" produced from palm oil. Its inclusion means that makeup adheres to the skin rather than being absorbed.

Mica General term used for a range of naturally occurring silicates. Mica gives a sparkle or pearlescence to cosmetics.

Parabens Broad spectrum preservative. Generally of vegetable or petroleum origin. Usage – approximately 4–6 drops per 100g product. Effective against fungus, yeast, bacteria, and mold.

Peach kernel oil Similar properties to apricot and almond oils; closer in texture to apricot.

Potato starch Prepared potato flour, which has emollient and gel-forming properties. Often an ingredient in baby powders. Used as a bulking and gel-forming agent in foundations.

Preservatives Parabens, germaben II, citrus seed extract.

Sandalwood oil (*Santalum album*) Strong antiseptic and soothing for the skin. Ability to preserve water within the skin without blocking pores.

Shea butter (Karite nut butter) Emollient, anti-irritant, slight sunscreen properties and is a natural cell regenerator.

Soy wax Naturally hardened soy with soft wax properties.

Stearic acid flakes A safe, universally used palm oil emulsifier, which is supplied in small, white flakes with a melting point similar to beeswax. Make sure you buy cosmetic-grade stearic acid flakes.

Talcum (Magnesium silicate) A natural mineral used in many makeup brands. Adheres well to the skin; produces density and slip. Care should be taken not to inhale dust.

Vitamin E oil (Tocopherol) Healing ingredient and antioxidant. Good for healthy cell regeneration and moisturizing.

Water Purified water should be used in skin-care cosmetics. Water is the primary ingredient in cosmetics that require preserving because it easily forms mold and carries bacteria.

Witch hazel Natural extract used as an astringent in skin-care cosmetics. Soothing and non-drying. Natural addition for toners for oil-rich skin.

Xanthan gum Thickener and stabilizer in emulsions.

NOTE: Metric measurements of small quantities are far more accurate than standard measures, and have been used throughout. Most of the ingredients used are sold by metric weight or volume, and measuring equipment is widely available.

PIGMENTS AND FUN ADDITIONS

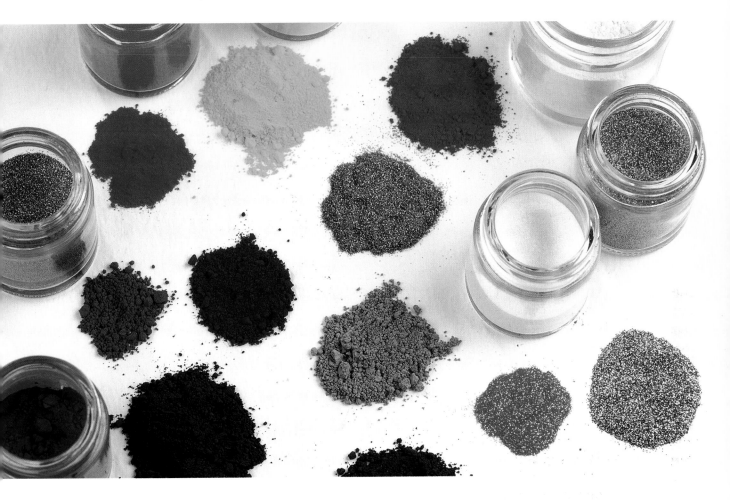

Pigments, powder colors, or dyes are found naturally in many herbs, flowers, and minerals. Their role in makeup recipes is to add color to the product and to the skin.
Dyes – soluble in either water or oil mediums, depending on the compound – are used to color the product, whereas pigments are used to color the skin or lashes (e.g., lipsticks and mascara are insoluble, yet may be dispersed rather than dissolved). Most cosmetics require less than five percent color in any product. Mixed to specific color matches from a variety of components, the finely milled powders are the backbone of the cosmetics industry. Commercially produced makeup formulations may contain varying degrees of 5, 10, or even 20 colors. To make things easier, I have used

ABOVE *Brightly colored ultramarines, rich, earthy iron oxides, and sparkling jewel tones are some of the colorants that you can use.*

a minimal number of colors in the recipes. However, with a little practice and experience, you will find yourself blending colors and ingredients to achieve more specialized and innovative products.

In this book I have tried as much as possible to use colors that are recommended worldwide as safe for use in makeup. However, inevitably, there are certain colors that are prohibited in some countries and not in others.

You should check carefully when buying, and if you are in any doubt, contact the relevant organization in your country. The Food and Drug Administration in the U.S. has approved a selection of colorants as suitable for safe use in food (F), drugs (D), and cosmetics (C). The FD&C colors are suitable for all three uses, but may have restrictions of usage, especially around the eyes and lips. D&C colors are for drug and cosmetic use, but again may have restrictions on their usage such as "external use only" or for wash-off products. **Pigment powders that are suitable for cosmetics and toiletries must never be ingested or inhaled. They should also be handled with care; otherwise, they can stain the skin.**

Each color has a CI (color index) number for industry recognition. **Pigments and dyes** are generally purchased in fine powder form. However, the powder is not fine enough in this state for making makeup. It is essential to pulverize them further in a mortar, using a pestle. Use a gentle action; the powder dust is very light. Take at least a minute or two to do this. Do not use a coffee grinder or food processor!

Created from a natural mineral, **titanium dioxide** is used in sunscreen, toothpaste, most powder makeup, and soap. It acts as a whitener and creates light-reflective microscopic spheres. It is used to give the appearance of smoothing and flattening wrinkles and removing dark circles under the eyes. In a concealer, titanium dioxide reflects light to lighten blemishes and therefore make darkened areas of skin appear more natural in tone. Titanium dioxide is the single most important color in all shades of makeup (regardless of skin tone) as it creates opacity. Opaque makeup can almost obliterate underlying skin colors and blemishes, and hide scars and pigment disorders. The color addition becomes less when the makeup needs to be translucent. Natural talcum forms the main base of translucent face powder.

Ultramarines used to be produced from china clay, but generally are now chemically reproduced. In a similar way to a potter painting clay that changes color when fired, ultramarines have specific fine minerals added, to change their color in the kiln, when dried. Ultramarines all have the same CI number; it is the specific additives that change the balance and therefore the color.

The **natural and nature-identical iron oxides** give wonderful color combinations, especially when mixed together or when combined with blacks and titanium dioxide to lighten and darken shades. A simple brown shade may be available from your supplier in a number of tones. The recipes indicate the brown shades you will require.

Another pigment group, known as **Lakes**, is made up of insoluble colors that give a light stain. These are usually used in lipsticks, nail polish, and face powders. When building up your color supplies, it is essential to have a little blue and green powder pigment in your selection. No, I am not expecting you to only make cobalt eye shadow, but a touch of blue in a reddish-toned makeup will soften it and make the finish more natural. Ivory and pale foundation will always be based on blue pigment.

Traditionally, the sparkle in makeup came from powdered fish scales, mother of pearl shell, and ultra-fine glass powder. Now we use fine mineral powders mixed with natural talcum or polyester sparkling flakes. **Glitter** and **mica** are micro capsules of fine sparkling metallic color. You must use fine-grade materials that are suitable for cosmetic use. Iridescent pigments are an "interference color." They are finely based on refracted and reflected light. Using titanium dioxide (white) in different micro-fine thicknesses changes the color intensity from its finest level – silvery white – through to yellows, reds, then when thicker, on to blues and greens. Note that some cosmetic-grade additives are not colorfast in warm or wet environments. For instance, a dry-mixed cosmetic glitter may be amazing, but in a lipstick, the heat from the molten waxes may have questionable effects! **If you are a contact lens wearer or have sensitive eyes, it is recommended that you do not use cosmetic glitter around the eye area.**

Domestic powdered herbs and spices should not be used in makeup as they can irritate the skin. You may find this a little odd as you've probably used soap that contains them, but makeup is designed to remain on the skin, unlike soap, which is a wash-off product. Likewise, candle wax dyes should not be used. **Basically, the rule is: always check that the product that you are buying is suitable for what you intend to use it for, and if you are in doubt, ask.**

SUITABLE COLORS FOR MAKEUP

NOTE: There are certain colors that are prohibited for use in makeup in some countries and not in others. You should check carefully when buying and if you are in any doubt, contact the relevant organization in your country.

Eyes
VIOLET/PURPLE
Manganese violet CI 77742
Ultramarine violet CI 77007
Red iron oxide (pink tone) CI 77491

BLUE
Ultramarine blue CI 77007
FD&C Blue no. I CI 42090

PINK
Ultramarine pink CI 77007

GREEN
D&C Green 5 CI 61570
Chromium oxide green CI 77288
Hydrated chromium oxide green CI 77289

WHITE
Titanium dioxide CI 77891

BLACK
Black iron oxide CI 77499 (external use)

DARK/BRICK RED
Red iron oxide CI 77491

MUSTARD/YELLOW
Yellow iron oxide CI 77492

Blended oxides – number followed by / 2 = additional yellow iron oxide
Number followed by / 9 = additional black iron oxide
Number followed by / I = additional red iron oxide
Example: Foundation base mid/dark tone red, yellow, and black iron oxide CI 77491/2/9

YELLOW
FD&C Yellow 5 CI 19140 water soluble

ORANGE/PEACH
FD&C Red 40 CI 16035
(F)D&C Yellow 6 CI 15985:1

Foundations
Oxides of black, red, and yellow. Shades of gray, brown, peach, and fawn. Generally mixed with permitted 5% addition of talcum by manufacturers.

SHADE TONING COLORS
Chromium oxide green – reduces redness in skin tone and foundation color.
Ultramarine blue (F)D&C Blue no. I – reduces redness, cools tone.

Lips
VIOLET/PLUM PINK
Manganese Violet CI 77742
D&C Red 33 CI 17200 (max. usage 3%)
BRIGHT PINK/RED
D&C Red 28 aluminum lake CI 45410:2

D&C Red 7 calcium lake CI 15850:1
D&C Red 22 aluminum lake CI 45380:3
D&C Red 30 CI 73360

PEACH/RED/PINK
D&C Red 6 CI 15850

TANGERINE/PEACH
(F)D&C Yellow 6 aluminum lake CI 15985:1

YELLOW
(F)D&C Yellow 5 aluminum lake CI 19140:1

BLUE
(F)D&C Blue no.I aluminum lake CI 42090:2

DILUTION PALER PINK
D&C Red 21 CI 45380:2
D&C Red 27 CI 45410:1

PLUM/RED/RED WINE/PINK
Carmine CI 75470 blue shade or yellow shade. (This color is produced from crushing shells of the cochineal insect. I have not used it.)

*Information sourced from Warner Jenkins Europe and Kingfisher Colours UK
Note: Ultramarines are permitted for use in lipsticks in the European Union.*

CONTAINERS AND STORAGE

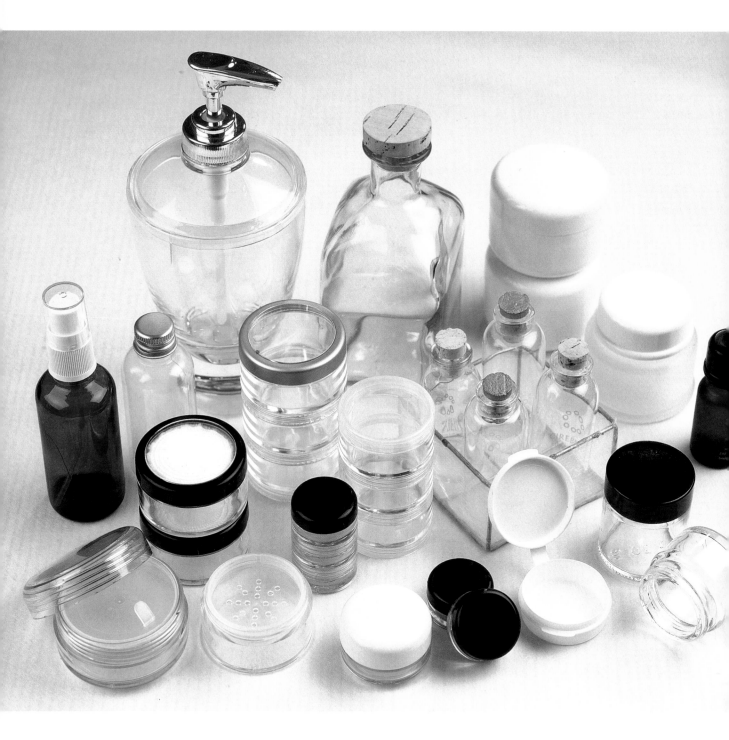

ABOVE *You can reuse old makeup containers or buy new ones (see Suppliers list on pages 94). Remember that they must be cleaned thoroughly and sterilized before use.*

I would not expect you to commission Lalique to design a bottle if you were making a perfume; likewise, it is not necessary to have a custom-designed eye shadow container either. The most convenient containers to use are old makeup containers (compacts, jars, lipsticks, etc.). Once you are hooked on making your own makeup, you will soon have exhausted supplies from all your friends and family. Note that you must not use discarded mascara tubes to put your homemade mascara in due to difficulties in removing any remaining mascara, sterilizing the inner tube, and the potential damage to the lining of the tube, which can harbor bacteria.

There are many "alternative" containers for the recipes. Start looking around your home, hardware stores, and accessory shops. You will start to see all sorts of storage containers in a whole new light! Plastic ring boxes, contact lens containers, and seven-day pill boxes will have a whole new range of uses. Even empty salt shakers are ideal to use for body glitter shakers. Lip colors and glosses can be stored in a small jar and applied with a brush. I will also show you how you can make a simple professional makeup stick (see page 36) and a lipstick mold (see page 47). This method is often used in color cosmetic formulation laboratories.

Whatever container you use, whether it is old or new, you must wash it in hot, soapy water and then sterilize it with boiling water or an appropriate sterilizing solution, such as isopropyl alcohol (see page 8). Hygiene must always be your first priority.

"Open" containers are not suitable to store makeup in because they can easily become contaminated with dust and foreign bodies which may damage the eyelids, lips, and skin. However, they can be useful when you are experimenting. I often use mineral water bottle tops when I'm trying out eye shadows and foundations. Artists' palettes are also useful if you're trying to come up with a complementary range of colors, since you can see all of the colors together.

When you make the recipes, any surplus base concentrates can be put into a closed container and stored in a cool, dark place for up to 12 weeks. Color powders, powder additives, and oils (if stored in a cool, dry place) can last 18 months or more.

You should label all your makeup, showing the date on which it was made, and you should discard the product after three months. The makeup is contaminated each time it is used – by the brush, sponge, finger, etc. that is put into it. The acid balance in your skin can change colors, and your natural skin oils can alter the fine balance of the recipes. Commercial makeup manufacturers understand this and pack their makeup full of preservatives and chemicals to prevent contamination and the damage that long-term storage can do, particularly to the containers the makeup is stored in. As a result of this, most of us think that it is fine to keep our purchased makeup for years, but it should also really be discarded after a few months, too.

Do not keep your homemade makeup in the refrigerator. The temperature drop can alter the delicate composition of the products, especially those containing waxes such as jojoba oil (which will solidify in the refrigerator and return to liquid at room temperature). Also, bacteria may be introduced into the makeup from spoiling food. It should just be stored in a cool, dry place.

Fresh makeup is more hygienic and needs fewer preservatives and unnatural additives than commercially manufactured makeup. It makes sense to create your makeup to coincide with the seasons and the clothes that you are wearing. A makeup that lasts the three months of one season can be economically updated when your mood, fashion, and the season change.

APPLICATORS

Applicators come in many shapes, sizes, and price ranges. It is more economical to buy good-quality brushes. They are less likely to shed their bristles as the head is fixed into a stem rather than just glued; therefore, they will last longer. A good brush is essential for the careful application of makeup. Fine-line brushes have a neat tapered tip, whereas the bolder, softer, fluffy blusher and foundation brushes are designed to hold the powders and have a gentle, plump surface. Lipstick, eye liner, and cream color all may be applied with a fine-line

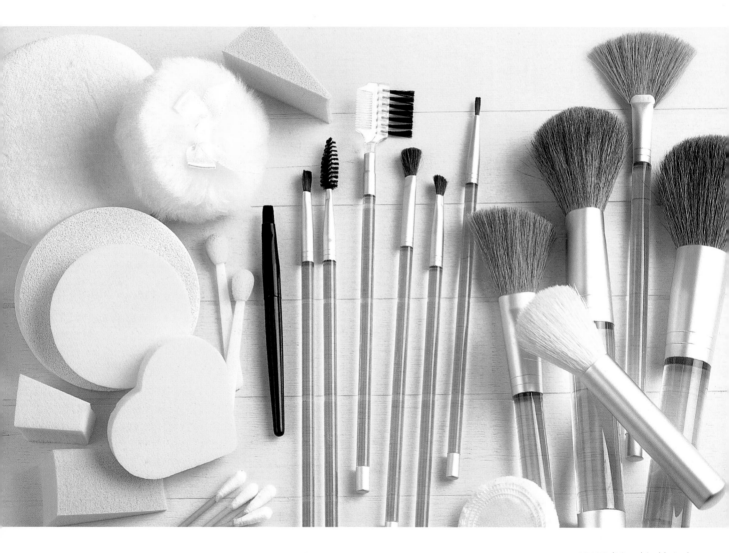

ABOVE *It is advisable to have a selection of brushes and applicators for each area of the face — eyes, lips, cheeks etc. The easiest way to do this is to buy a makeup brush kit.*

brush. A flatter, wedge-tipped brush can be used for filling in lip colors. It is more hygienic to use a brush for lipstick than applying straight from the lipstick itself. When applying blushers, load your soft brush and holding the handle down, shake the powder into the body of the bristles, tap the excess, and apply. This gives an even coating and prevents the need to keep returning the brush to your container. It is advisable to have a brush for each task, and most supermarkets, department stores, and pharmacies sell a selection or a makeup brush kit. Consider yourself an artist; every artist needs a selection of brushes.

Soft sponges made of latex are suitable for foundations, color application, and blending concealers. They are easy to clean and sterilize, are available in wedges, pads, and compact puffs, and may be used dry or damp. A little clean, warm, previously boiled water poured on the sponge and then squeezed until almost dry is the best way to apply makeup with a damp applicator. You can then strengthen eye colors, strongly define lines, and apply a creamy foundation with a sheer effect.

I like disposable foam applicators and cotton swabs. When applying eye makeup, use one cotton swab for each eye. You can use one side for dark and one side for paler colors. Apply the paler colors first, shade with the darker tones, then blend. This way, you will never introduce any contamination into your makeup or onto yourself. Discard after use.

Good hygiene is of paramount importance when storing and using brushes and applicators for makeup. Clean, makeup free brushes should be kept in a wrap or pencil-style case, separate from your makeup. I like to spray a little toner onto clean brushes to remove grease deposits and rinse a second time. Baby bottle sterilizing solution is an ideal way to make sure that foam pads and applicators are clean. Rinse in running water, dry, and store. Although cleansing bristle brushes in very hot or boiling water is a good cleaning method, it can also soften the glues keeping the bristles in place. If you wish to clean your brushes this way, place only the tip in water, not the stem or barrel.

SAFETY GUIDELINES

• Wax has a low melting point, and if it gets too hot, it can burst into flames just like cooking oil. Treat it with respect and never leave a pan unattended. Use a very low heat; watch the wax grains melt. As soon as they have melted and you have clear liquid (which only takes a few seconds), the wax is at a working temperature.

• If wax catches fire, smother the flames with a damp dishtowel or kitchen fire blanket. Do NOT attempt to quench the flames with water because this will splash burning wax everywhere.

• Always use a thermometer when heating wax so you know that it is not getting too hot.

• If you spill hot wax on your skin, immediately hold the area under the cold running faucet. Hot wax rarely scalds if you keep it at the temperature required.

• Use oven gloves or some kind of hand protection when handling hot bowls, beakers, etc., that do not have handles and when pouring hot liquids.

• Keep pets and young children away from the area where you are making your makeup.

• All containers must be washed and sterilized before use (see page 17).

• Label your makeup to show the date on which it was made and discard after three months.

• Do not allow anyone else to use your makeup.

• Wash and clean all of your applicators regularly.

• Only use products that are suitable for use in cosmetics – if in doubt, check with the supplier.

• It is recommended that you test each product that you make on a small area of skin on your inner forearm first, before using it fully. Leave overnight. If any sensitivity occurs, the makeup recipe is unsuitable for you.

• The makeup made using the recipes in this book is for personal use only, it must not be sold.

EYES

Eye makeup should be used to enhance your eyes – in terms of their color and shape – and not just to provide decoration (except for fun party makeup, of course). Keep your "evening eyes" for glamorous occasions and have a more natural look during the day. In this chapter there are recipes for eye shadows, eye liners, and mascara in a variety of colors to suit all skin tones, so you'll find something you like. Once you've gotten used to handling the materials and become familiar with the color pigments, experiment to create your very own color.

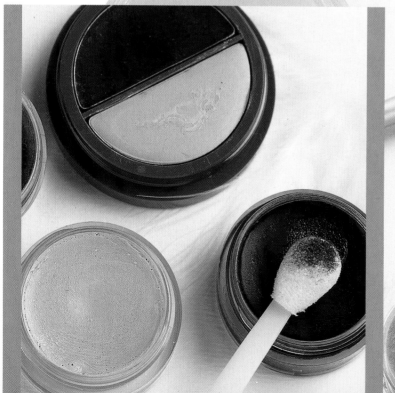

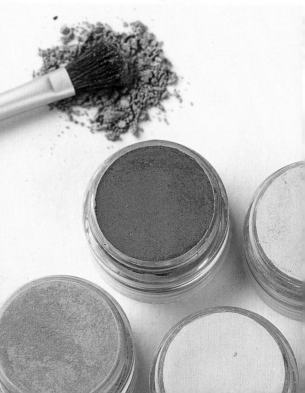

EYE SHADOWS

Powdered eye shadow is designed to be applied from a compact or container using a brush or sponge applicator. The intensity of color can be increased by using a damp applicator. In addition to compacted eye shadows, I've included some recipes for crème eye shadows and makeup sticks. The method for each group of eye shadows is the same; the only thing that you need to change to get different colors is the pigment powders. Once you gain confidence in handling the pigments, experiment to create your own color palettes.

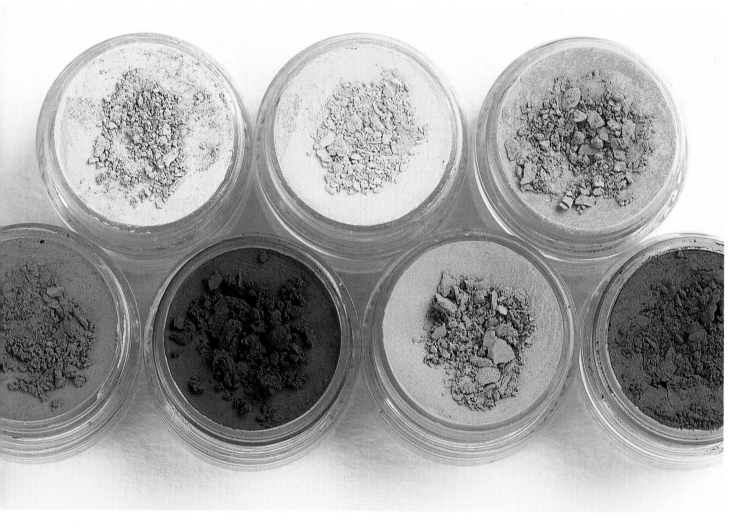

DUO POWDERS

These powder shadows are light and dark tones of the same color. I've given recipes for brown, lilac, and blue shades. When making the recipes, I would recommend you add the jojoba oil from a dropper bottle as it is much easier than measuring with a spoon. Keep any reserved base for future projects. Because the amounts of some ingredients used in the recipes are so small, it is sometimes necessary to make more of some parts than is immediately required.

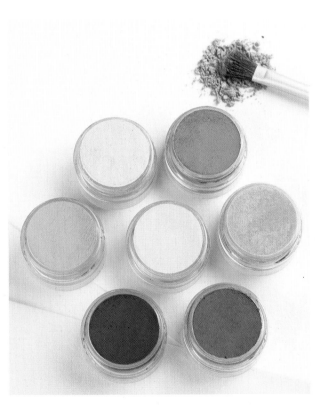

LEFT *Choose colors to match your eyes and the shade of your skin. This will enhance your features rather than dominate them with color.*

ABOVE *Filling your container to the brim makes the powder easier to compact and gives an even surface.*

Basic Matte Powder Eye Shadow

There are two stages to making the basic powder eye shadow. Part 1 is the base concentrate. In Part 2 you use a portion of your base concentrate and by mixing in the appropriate colors, the desired shade will be achieved.

Makes 3–4 x 10g jars

INGREDIENTS
PART 1
2 tsp talcum
1 tsp cornstarch
½ tsp magnesium stearate

PART 2
1 tsp jojoba oil
½ tsp talcum
¼ tsp cornstarch

EQUIPMENT
Measuring spoons
Bowl
Teaspoon
Screw-cap jar (for excess powder base)
Pestle and mortar
Dropper bottle
Eye makeup containers

PART 1
1 Place all the dry ingredients in a bowl and blend.

PART 2
2 Put 1 teaspoon of the base concentrate (Part 1 above) into the mortar. Add 10 drops of jojoba oil and, using the pestle, mix until the oil is fully absorbed.
3 Add a further 1–2 drops of jojoba oil and, using the pestle again, mix until fully absorbed.
4 Place the additional talcum and cornstarch into the mortar and mix. You can now add the color pigments.

LUSCIOUS CHOCOLATE CARAMEL CREAM

Pigment colors
(Brown) iron oxide – oak tone
(Brown) iron oxide – walnut tone
(Red) iron oxide – peach tone
Titanium dioxide – white
Yellow iron oxide (optional)

Tip
Before using any pigments, "work" them in a mortar with a pestle to get rid of any lumps or air pockets. This will prevent your makeup from being streaky or rough.

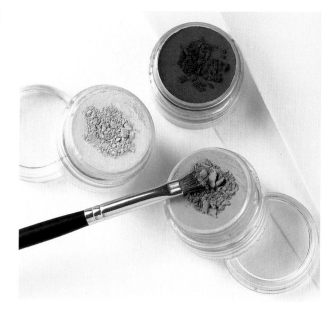

CHOCOLATE

1 Add a matchhead of both brown iron oxides to powder mix made in Part 2 (see page 23).

2 Mix well with pestle to remove all microscopic lumps and air-filled pockets of powder. This usually takes a minute or two.

3 Add ¼ matchhead (a tiny amount) of red iron oxide. Mix well.

4 Add a further matchhead of titanium dioxide. This is always quite lumpy and needs careful preparation when incorporating into the brown mix. When you are happy with the brown tone, you may wish to add a little more brown, red, or yellow, depending on your color choice.

5 Add 2–3 drops of jojoba oil and mix thoroughly. Add a further drop of jojoba oil and repeat.

6 If you want to just use this basic color shade on its own, put the eye shadow into a container and press to compact (see page 25). However, if you wish to make a contrasting shade, you will need to divide this basic color into two and use half of it to make Caramel (see right); if you also want to make a third highlighter color, Cream (see right), divide the basic color into three.

CARAMEL

1 Put the appropriate quantity of Chocolate eye shadow into your mortar (see step 6 below left).

2 Add ¼ teaspoon of talcum, ¼ teaspoon cornstarch, ½ matchhead of yellow iron oxide, and ¼ matchhead of red iron oxide (peach tone). Use the pestle to mix to a tan shade. Add a little titanium dioxide if it is too yellow.

3 Add 2–4 drops of jojoba oil and use the pestle to mix until all of the oil is absorbed and the color is uniform and has no streaks. If the color is too dark, adjust it with a little more titanium dioxide.

4 Compact the powder into a container (see page 25).

CREAM

1 In the mortar mix together the remaining Chocolate eye shadow, ½ teaspoon of base concentrate (see Part 1 page 23), and ¼ teaspoon of titanium dioxide. Carefully mix for 1–2 minutes.

2 Add 2–4 drops of jojoba oil and incorporate fully. Add a drop or two more if required.

3 Press the powder into a container to compact (see page 25).

Beauty tip

Although these eye shadows are duo (two) color recipes, I have included a third, lighter tone for the browns to make a highlighting color to coordinate with your palette. Wear the highlighter below the brow line and on the middle of the lid to create a lifting effect.

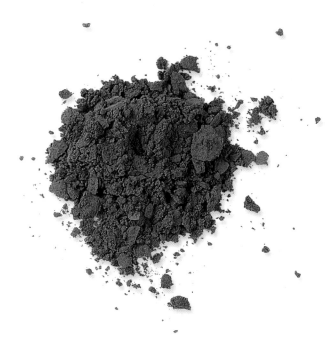

COMPACTING EYE SHADOWS INTO A CONTAINER

Although matte shadows can be used in powdered form, you will probably want to compact them into a container for ease of storage and to give a flatter surface for visual appeal. However, don't expect to achieve the same kind of results as you see in purchased makeup. To compact these products so perfectly, they are pounded with immense pressure using high-tech machinery.

Method 1
This is the easiest and quickest way of compacting eye shadow.

1 Fill the container with the loose powder. Cover the surface of the powder with plastic wrap.
2 Using the tip of your thumb or index finger, press the powder into the container. If you want to include two colors, fill half of the pot with each color.
3 Press firmly to compact, working neatly from the outer edges to the center and back. Remove wrap.

Method 2
This method compacts the powder to a greater degree.

1 Fill the container with powder. Find a clean coin or counter disk (about the size of your container) and double-wrap it in plastic wrap. For a rectangular or square container, use a small piece of plastic or smooth wood, and wrap as above.
2 Place on the surface of the eye shadow and press down on it firmly. This will compact the shadow and give it a smooth surface.

Method 3
Using a rubber stamp creates an attractive impression on the surface of the shadow. For hygiene reasons keep some stamps specifically for this task. Do not use stamps that you have used for any other purpose.

1 Fill the container with the eye shadow powder. Cover the surface of the powder with plastic wrap. Find a rubber stamp or seal of a suitable size. Flatten the surface of the shadow with your index finger.
2 Remove the wrap. Align the stamp over the powder and then press it down firmly on the surface. Be sure not to move the stamp or the container.
3 Carefully lift the stamp off the surface in one clean movement without twisting.

PRETTY VIOLET AND LAVENDER

Pigment colors
Ultramarine violet
Ultramarine blue
Ultramarine pink
Titanium dioxide
Red iron oxide (deep mahogany tone)

VIBRANT VIOLET

1 Repeat Part 2 (see page 23). Blend together ¼ teaspoon ultramarine violet, a few grains of ultramarine pink, and a tiny amount of titanium dioxide. Mix well to create a strong shade. A deeper, blue-toned violet needs a few grains of ultramarine blue.

2 Compact half of this powder into a container (see page 25) and use the other half to make the lighter Lovely Lavender shade (see below).

LOVELY LAVENDER

1 Place remaining Vibrant Violet powder into a mortar.

2 Add ¼ teaspoon titanium dioxide, ¼ teaspoon ultramarine pink, ½ teaspoon base concentrate (see Part 1, page 23). Mix until lavender tone is achieved.

3 To make a deeper pink tone, add a little more ultramarine pink or a few grains of red iron oxide and make sure the colors are totally blended.

4 Add 2–4 drops of jojoba oil. Add a drop more if you think the mix is too dry. Compact (see page 25).

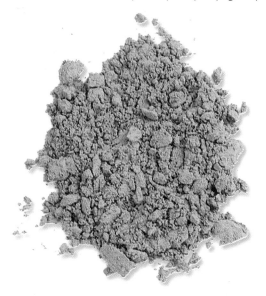

GREENERY

Pigment colors
Sage green — chromium oxide green
(External use) brown iron oxide (walnut tone)
Ultramarine blue
Yellow iron oxide (fawn tone)
Titanium dioxide

OLIVE

1 Repeat Part 2 (see page 23). Add ¼ teaspoon sage green, ½ matchhead (external use) brown iron oxide (walnut tone), and a few grains of ultramarine blue (use very sparingly). Mix thoroughly.

2 Compact half of this powder into a container and use the other half to make Soft Palm (below).

SOFT PALM

1 Place remaining Olive into a mortar, along with ¼ teaspoon fawn yellow iron oxide and ¼ teaspoon titanium dioxide. Mix well.

2 Compact into a container (see page 25).

Beauty tip
Greens can be blue, brown, or yellow in tone. Soft greens, teal, and olive tones look subtle on the eyelids, with a slightly darkened area shaded into your socket line and a paler color highlighted under the brow. The highlighter color also looks effective when worn on your eyelids with a darker green line defining the socket. For softer, subtler greens than those shown, use more titanium dioxide and hydrated chromium oxide.

RIGHT *Greenery — soft, natural greens can be worn all year round, with shading to complement warm or cool colors.*

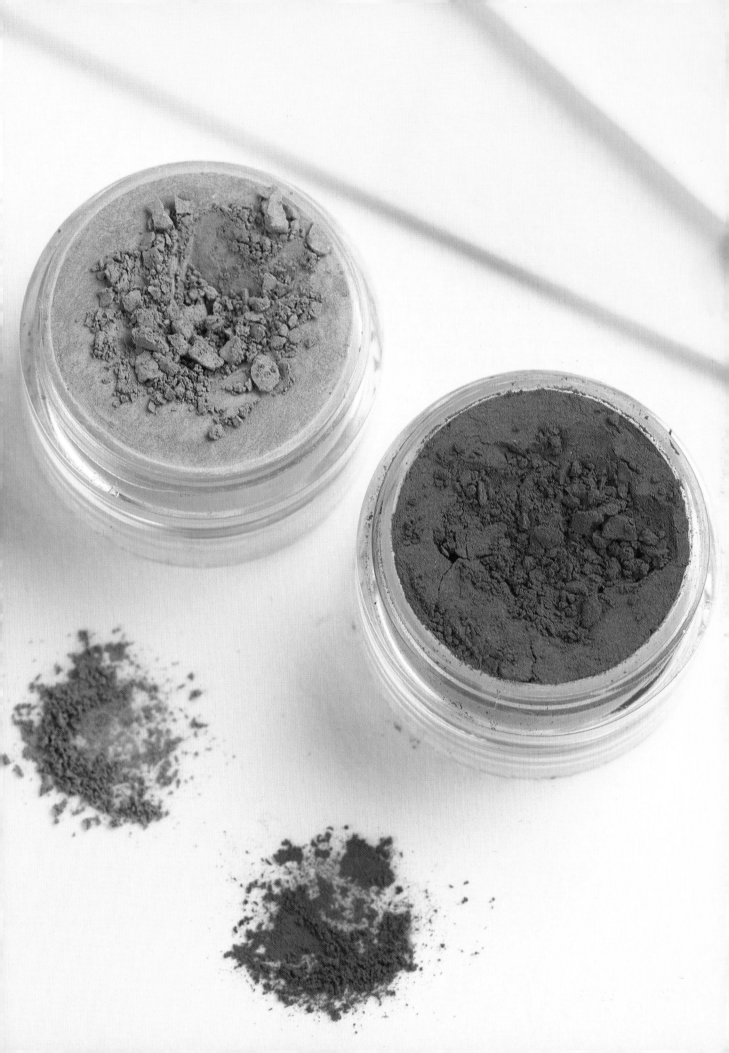

FROSTED SHADOWS

These crème shadows, in light and dark tones, are suitable for application above the eyelid. To create the frosty sparkle in the colors, I have added mineral sparkle. You must make sure that you use this or cosmetic-grade glitter; other products can scratch, damage, and irritate the eyes. I've given the basic instructions for creating two or three shades for each color group, but feel free to experiment and create a palette of lighter and darker tones.

Basic Frosted Crème Eye Shadow

This is your uncolored crème shadow base.

Makes enough for one color group

INGREDIENTS

PART 1

2 tsp talcum

1 tsp cornstarch

½ tsp magnesium stearate

PART 2

1 tbsp jojoba oil

1g carnauba wax

1g cosmetic beeswax

EQUIPMENT

Measuring spoons

Pestle and mortar

Teaspoon

Screw-cap jar

Kitchen scales

Double boiler

Thermometer

Heat-resistant beaker

Coffee stirrer

Eye makeup containers

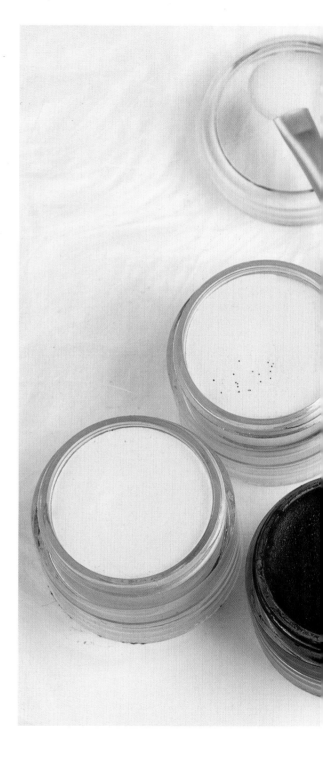

PART 1

1 Place all the ingredients in the mortar and blend well with a spoon. Put in a screw-cap jar.

PART 2

2 Put the jojoba oil and waxes into the upper pan of the double boiler and put hot water in the lower pan. Heat gently until the wax melts and the oil and wax form a clear liquid. Do not exceed 160°F when heating.

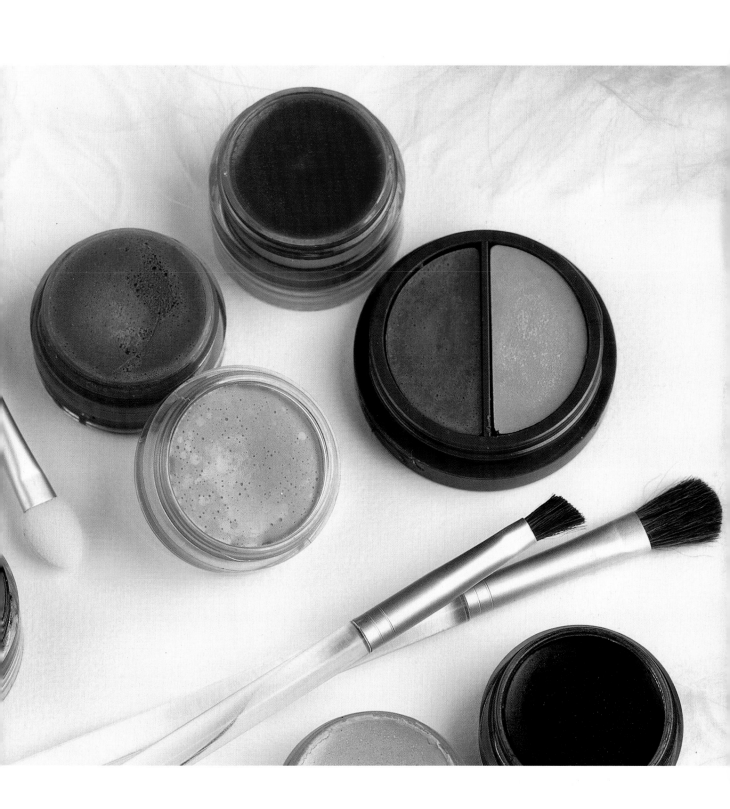

3 Remove from the heat and mix Part I with Part 2. This makes enough to use as a base for one group of colors. You can now add the colors of your choice (see pages 30–34).

ABOVE *Double-sectioned containers and small stacking jars make an easy storage solution for light and dark colors that work in harmony together. Try subtle and strong shades together for a dramatic evening or party effect.*

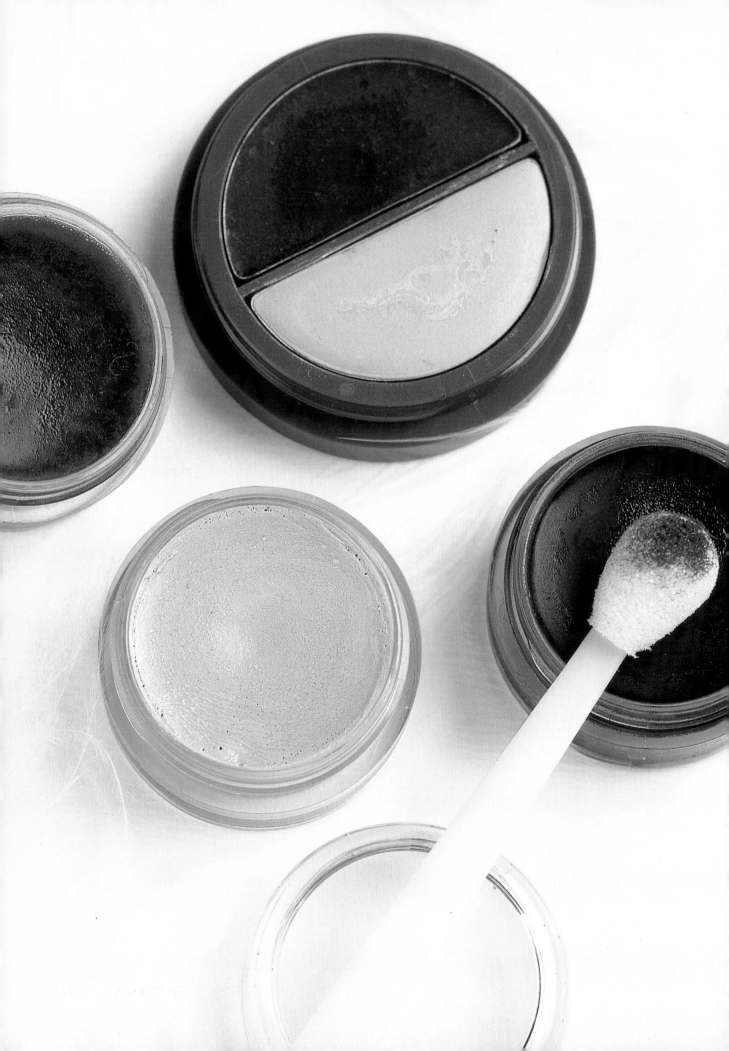

BLUES – DARK TO SKY

Pigment colors/additions

Ultramarine blue

(External use) black iron oxide

Titanium dioxide

Pearl mica

Tip

Oil-based makeup can have wonderful contrasting effects with powder and shimmering eye shadows.

SHIMMERING COBALT BLUE

1 Make a quantity of Basic Frosted Crème Eye Shadow (see pages 28–29).

2 Place ¼ teaspoon of ultramarine blue, a few grains of (external use) black iron oxide and titanium dioxide, and ¼ teaspoon (add a little more for a softer shade) pearl mica in a mortar and blend together with a pestle. Transfer to a heat-resistant beaker.

3 Reheat the crème base in the double boiler if it has solidified and add to the pigment powders, blending thoroughly with a spoon. It may solidify or form lumps, but keep mixing, and reheat if necessary. The mixture can be reheated many times.

4 Pour half of the Shimmering Cobalt Blue crème shadow mixture into containers and let it set in a cool room for 1–2 hours. Keep the other half to use as a base from which to mix more colors.

LEFT *This range of blue colors can be used to create a dramatic effect for the evening.*

DARK BLUE HUE

1 In a heat-resistant beaker, mix a matchhead (you can use slightly more or less depending on how dark you want the color to be) of (external use) black iron oxide powder with half of the remaining Shimmering Cobalt Blue crème (left, reheat as necessary).

2 Pour into containers and let it set in a cool room for 1–2 hours.

PALE SKY BLUES

1 Mix ¼ teaspoon titanium dioxide and ½ teaspoon pearl mica in a mortar and use a pestle to disperse any lumps (however small). Transfer to a heat-resistant beaker.

2 Reheat the remaining Shimmering Cobalt Blue crème (see left), remove from the heat, and add to the powder mix. Mix thoroughly with a spoon; then pour into containers.

3 Leave it to set in a cool room for 1–2 hours.

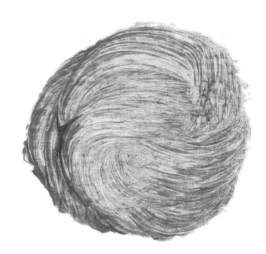

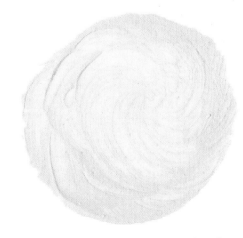

PURPLE SKY-BLUE PINK

Pigment colors/additions
+/- matchhead ultramarine violet
+/- matchhead ultramarine pink
(External use) black iron oxide
Ultramarine blue
Titanium dioxide
⅛ tsp pearl mica

1 Make a quantity of Basic Frosted Crème Eye Shadow
(see pages 28–29).
2 Prepare each pigment separately in a mortar, using the
pestle to eliminate any lumps. Put the ultramarine violet
and ultramarine pink into separate heat-resistant
beakers. These two basic colors can be varied by adding
a few grains of the following: external-use black iron
oxide to darken; ultramarine blue to give them a more
blue tone; black and blue for navy/plum tones; or
titanium dioxide for a deeper, more opaque shade or a
lighter/pastel version.
3 Mix half of the crème base into each color and then
add half of the mica to each.
4 Pour into containers and let them set in a cool room
for 1–2 hours.

Tip
*I've only given instructions to make two colors, but
obviously you can make as many tonal variations as you
like to create a palette of colors; just use the crème
base, colors, and mica proportionally.*

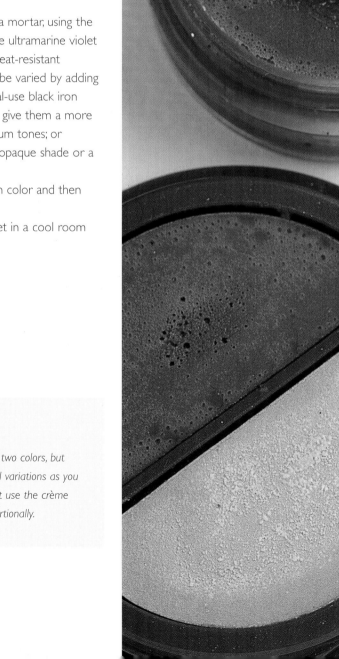

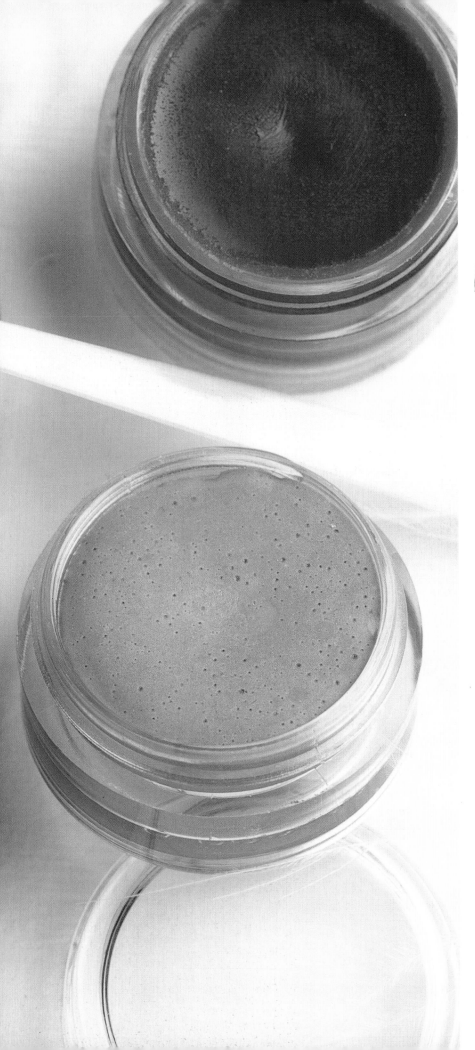

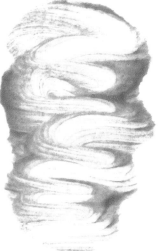

LEFT *Natural pearl mica is added to create a light-reflective finish. When applied, it creates the illusion of widening the eyes.*

VAMP EYES

Pigment colors/additions

¼ tsp (external use) black iron oxide

Pinch ultramarine blue (optional)

¼ tsp titanium dioxide

Pinch pearl mica

Pinch silver cosmetic-grade glitter (optional; must be
suitable for use in eye shadows)

BLACK AS NIGHT

1 Make a quantity of Basic Frosted Crème Eye Shadow
(see pages 28–29; half will be used for this color and half
for Light of the Moon, see right).

2 Work the black iron oxide in the mortar, using the
pestle. Add the ultramarine blue to create a deep
midnight-blue color. Transfer to a heat-resistant beaker.

3 Add half of the crème base (reheat as necessary) to
the powder.

4 Pour into containers and let it set for 1–2 hours in a
cool room.

LIGHT OF THE MOON

1 Place the titanium dioxide and pearl mica in the mortar
and work with the pestle. Transfer to a heat-resistant
beaker.

2 Mix the prepared powder pigments with the remaining
crème base (you may need to reheat this slightly if it has
started to solidify).

3 Add a pinch of silver glitter and stir it in with a coffee
stirrer.

4 Pour into containers and let them set in a cool room for
1–2 hours.

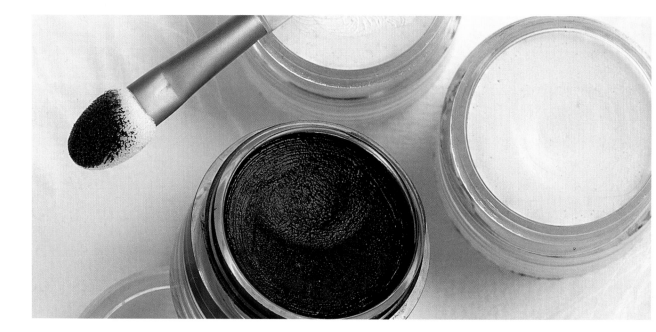

ABOVE *Dress to enhance the
effect of your dramatic makeup.
Use your color with careful
attention to detail to create a
stunning effect.*

ℬeauty tip

*Vamp colors can range from stunning dark plums
to midnight blues to dense blacks. You can also make
tones of gray or add a touch of blue or violet to enhance
the moody effect.*

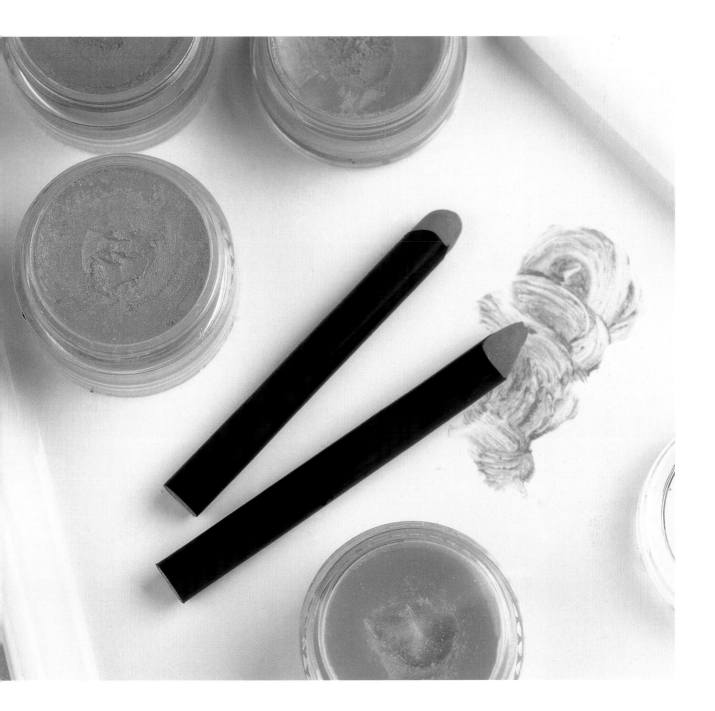

FUNKY FUN EYES

This is an easy way to make fun, party, and special-effects makeup that is suitable for use on the eyes, face, and body. You can make any color, but I like to create bold shades. They are easy to remove – use a gentle cleanser for the face or mild soap and water for the body. You can put these colors into jars, or you can make them in the form of color sticks (see page 36). If you store the color in a jar, it should be applied with a foam applicator or brush.

ABOVE *Decoration does not stop at your eyes. These colors can be used on your lips, cheeks, shoulders, arms, and legs.*

Wax Base

Makes 3–4 x 2½-in straws or 2 x 10g jars

INGREDIENTS
1 tbsp jojoba oil
½ tsp cosmetic beeswax
½ tsp crushed carnauba wax

EQUIPMENT
Measuring spoons
Double boiler
Thermometer
Stirring spoon
Kitchen scales
Pestle and mortar
Heat-resistant beakers
Eye makeup containers

1 Put the ingredients into the upper pan of the double boiler and put hot water in the lower pan. Heat until the wax is just melting (do not exceed 160°F).

SHOCKING PINK

Pigment colors/additions
¼ tsp FD&C red 40 or D&C red 33
Pinch talcum
Pinch cornstarch
1g titanium dioxide

1 Mix all of the pigment colors and additions together in a mortar. Mix well, pressing out all of the lumps and air pockets. Transfer to a heat-resistant beaker.
2 You need to use half a quantity of Wax Base (see left; you could try making half a quantity of Wax Base, but the measurements would be tiny and it would be difficult to make accurately). Reheat if it has started to solidify. Quickly mix the powders into the wax base.
3 Carefully pour the mixture into containers. Protect your hands as the mixture will be hot. Reserve a little of the mixture for topping up.
4 Leave to harden for 1-2 hours. There may be a little shrinkage, so just reheat the reserved color mixture and top up.

MAKING COLOR STICKS

These sticks are really easy to make and are a unique and fun way of storing your homemade makeup. You can sharpen them to a soft point using a makeup sharpener and then apply them to your skin. Use a light touch so as not to scratch your skin.

EQUIPMENT
Drinking straws (the widest you can find) cut into 2½-in
*   lengths*
Aluminum foil cut into 3 x ¾-in pieces
Ramekin or dish filled with flour
Small heat-resistant measuring cup with pouring lip
Make-up sharpener

1 Take a length of straw and wrap the foil around one end. Leave enough foil overhanging the end of the straw that you can twist it to close off the end.
2 Gently push the foil-wrapped straw (closed end first) into the dish filled with flour so that it is standing upright.
3 Once you have your mixture ready, carefully pour it into the straw sticks. Protect your hands as the wax mixture will be hot. Reserve a little for topping up.
4 Leave to harden for 1–2 hours. There may be a little shrinkage, so just reheat the reserved color mixture in a double boiler and top up. Leave to set again.
5 Peel off the foil and sharpen to a gentle point. Your stick is now ready to use. Wrap in plastic wrap or place in a plastic food bag to keep the tip clean.

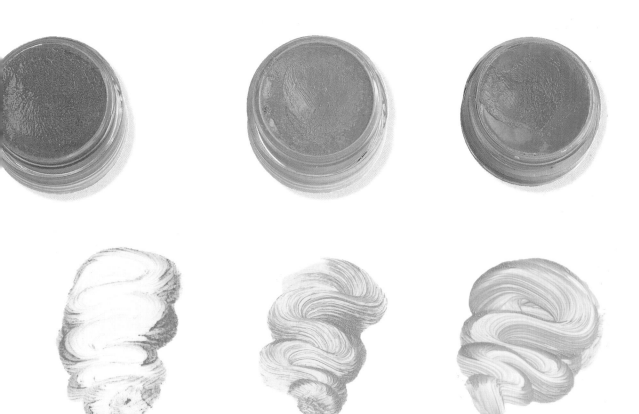

GOLDEN SPARKLE

Pigment colors/additions
Pinch FD&C yellow 5
¼ tsp yellow iron oxide
¼ tsp pearl mica
Pinch gold cosmetic-grade glitter (must be suitable for use in eye shadows)

1 Mix the pigment colors and the mica together in a mortar. Press out any lumps and air pockets using the pestle. Transfer to a heat-resistant beaker.
2 Reheat half a quantity of Wax Base (see page 36). Quickly add to the powder mix and stir, then add the glitter and stir. Pour into containers; protect your hands as the mixture will be hot. Reserve a little for topping up.
3 Leave to harden for 1–2 hours. The mixture may have shrunk a little; if it has, top up with the reserved mixture.

ABOVE *You can make this party makeup in wild and wacky colors. You'll certainly be the center of attention!*

EYE LINER

Eye liner can be worn as a soft, shadow line or a fine, strong, painted color line. This wax-based eye liner is for soft lines; add double the amount of carnauba wax if you require a harder edge. You can store your eye liner in a jar and apply it with a brush, or make Color Sticks (see page 36). You need half a quantity of wax base (see Part 1 below) for each color.

BROWN-EYED GIRL

Makes 3 x 10g jars

INGREDIENTS
PART 1
1 tbsp jojoba oil
½ tsp cosmetic beeswax
½ tsp crushed carnauba wax
¼ tsp stearic acid flakes

PART 2
Pigment colors: ¼ tsp brown iron oxide (dark nut tone),
* pinch (external use) black iron oxide*
¼ tsp talcum
¼ tsp cornstarch
¼ tsp magnesium stearate
1-2 drops germaben II

EQUIPMENT
Measuring spoons
Double boiler
Thermometer
Stirring spoon
Dropper bottle or pipette
Pestle and mortar
Heat-resistant beaker
Eye makeup containers

PART 1
1 Put the ingredients in the upper pan of the double boiler and hot water into the lower pan. Heat until the wax is just melting (do not exceed 160°F). This is the wax base of the eye liner. Set aside.

PART 2
2 Place all of the ingredients in a mortar. Mix well and press out all of the lumps and air pockets using the pestle. Transfer to a heat-resistant beaker.
3 Reheat half of the Part 1 wax base in the double boiler and quickly mix with the Part 2 powder.
4 Pour into a container; protect your hands as the mixture will be hot. Let it set in a cool room for 1–2 hours.

BLUE-BLACK

Pigment colors
¼ tsp black iron oxide
(+/-) matchhead ultramarine blue (depending on how
* blue or black you want the color to be)*

PART 1
1 Follow the ingredients and instructions for Part 1 (left).

PART 2
2 Follow the ingredients and instructions for Part 2 (left), but use the pigment colors specified above instead.

WHITE ICICLES

Pigment colors/additions
½ tsp titanium dioxide
¼ tsp pearl mica

PART 1
1 Follow the ingredients and instructions for Part 1 (left).

PART 2
2 Follow the ingredients and instructions for Part 2 (left), but use the pigment colors/additions specified above instead.

Beauty tip
This unusual white eye liner looks particularly striking on those with dark skin.

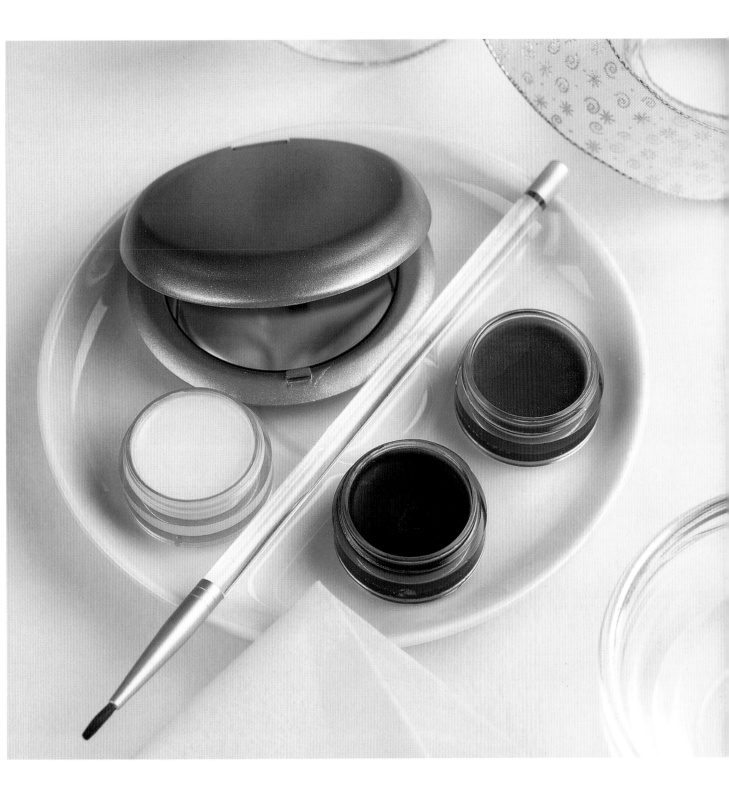

ABOVE *Eye liner can be applied directly to the skin to create the illusion of changing the shape of your eyes or used over eye shadow to line the eyelashes.*

KOHL

In India, kohl is traditionally made by mixing lampblack (the soot produced from burning oil or gas) with animal fat. In other Asian countries it is made by blackening the edges of a ceramic or metal dish with a candle flame in order to produce soot. When there is a sufficient build up of the greasy candle soot, oil such as castor oil is added and blended to produce waxy kohl. Needless to say, none of the kohl made commercially is made in this way, and neither is my homemade kohl.

Makes 10g of product

INGREDIENTS

2 tsp castor oil
½ tsp cosmetic beeswax
Pinch stearic acid flakes
¼ tsp (external use) black iron oxide
2 drops germaben II or liquid parabens

EQUIPMENT

Measuring spoons
Double boiler
Stirring spoon
Pestle and mortar
Heat-resistant beaker
Small containers

1 Put the castor oil, beeswax, and stearic acid flakes into the upper pan of the double boiler and put hot water into the lower pan. Heat until the wax just starts to melt (do not exceed 140°F).
2 Work the black iron oxide in a mortar with a pestle. Transfer to a heat-resistant beaker and carefully add the oil and wax mixture. Add preservative and mix well.
3 Pour into small containers. Leave in a cool place to set.

ABOVE *Use a cotton swab or a brush to apply the kohl. Apply to the inner rim of the eyelid, just inside the lash line, and draw into a slight point at the outer corners of the eyes.*

RIGHT *You can make mascara in any color that you want, even vibrant orange as shown here. Check that the color pigments you choose are suitable for use around the eyes.*

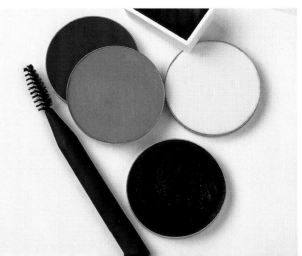

MASCARA

Preservatives are essential in this recipe so NEVER attempt to omit them. Do not keep the mascara for more than three months. Apply with a flat brush. Although this is not a waterproof recipe, it will give a natural sheen to the lashes.

Makes 20g of product
(most commercial mascaras weigh between 3–7g)

INGREDIENTS

Total of 2–3 matchheads very finely ground pigments (see color suggestions opposite)
½ tsp carnauba wax
½ tsp soy wax
¼ tsp stearic acid flakes
1 tsp vitamin E oil
Few drops lemon juice
2 drops germaben II or liquid parabens

EQUIPMENT

Pestle and mortar
Measuring spoons
Double boiler
Thermometer
Juice squeezer
Dropper bottle or pipette
Stirring spoon
Pestle and mortar
New mascara tubes

1 Work your chosen color pigments with the pestle in the mortar until ultra fine. Set aside.

2 Put the waxes into the upper pan of the double boiler and put hot water into the lower pan. Heat gently until the wax is just melted (do not exceed 160°F).

3 Add the remaining ingredients and stir until liquid appears clear.

4 With the boiler still on a gentle heat, add the pigments and stir until incorporated.

5 Carefully pour into a new mascara tube.

Tip
A soft, creamy mascara can be made by substituting the soy wax with petroleum jelly.

BLACK AND BROWN

To create black, brown, and myriad brown/black shades follow the instructions below. For a strong black, use a single (external use) black iron oxide in your formula. For brown mascara, simply choose the brown iron oxide shade you prefer and blend it with a few grains of black (for opacity).

To create brown/black shades, discount a little black and add brown iron oxide.

BLUES

Starting with a black base and little pinches of ultramarine blue, carefully blend your powders to a dark blue tone. To make a stronger, brighter blue, add more blue and less black.

WHITE

For partywear, add titanium dioxide with a pinch or two of white pearl mica. This will make a clear white product. Apply mascara carefully.

Beauty tips
Use a brush with a lash comb and brush combination. Carefully pre-cleanse your eyelashes. The lashes harbor dust and germs that should be removed before application. Comb the lashes to separate them and remove loose hair. Carefully apply a fine layer of color cream to the lashes and let it set. Repeat a second time if required.

LIPS

This chapter will encourage newcomers to lipstick to try gentle colors and regular wearers to develop colors to suit their taste. There is a fun section called Lips to Shock! – wait until you see the colors. The recipes are all made with natural oils and waxes, and are designed to enrich and moisturize the lips. There is also a wonderful natural lip balm recipe. All of these recipes are easy to make, and can be firmed into a lipstick tube or fill a jar. Have fun, be creative, and you will find the cost involved is a fraction of store prices.

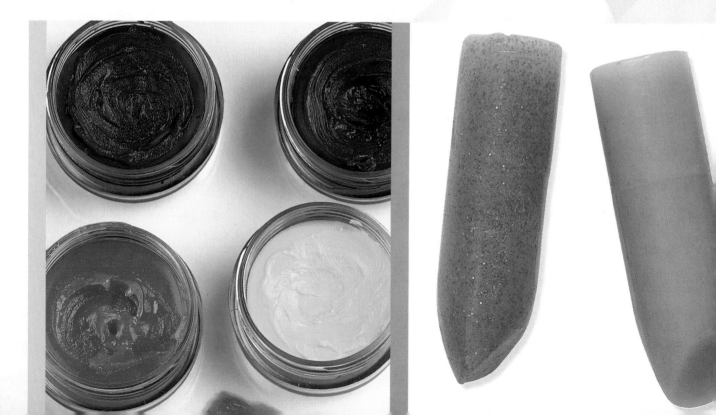

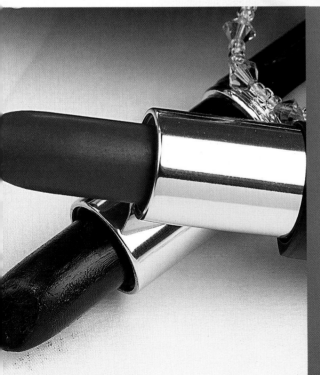

LIPSTICK

Finding the perfect lipstick color is almost impossible. How many lipsticks do you have in your makeup bag that you never use? Making your own lipstick is the answer, as you can create that elusive color just for you, and it is great fun. Customized precision molds carefully crafted to make a seamfree "bullet" of wax-based color are available, but they are expensive. However, you don't have to have one of these to make your own lipstick. Specialized suppliers can sometimes provide a single plastic mold, or there is a very simple way of creating your own mold using little more than a pen or dowel and some aluminum foil.

BELOW *Kiss gloss colors can be a transparent gloss or a sheer hint of color. They can also be used over stronger color to give added shine.*

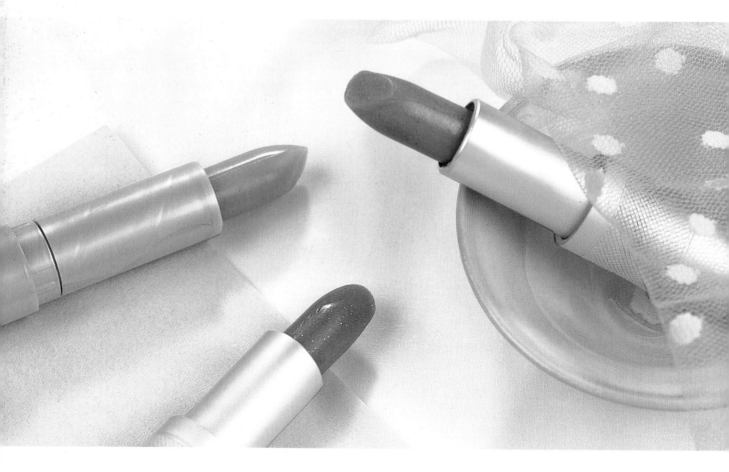

KISS GLOSS COLORS

These colors give the lips a light, glossy effect and a tint of color. These are colors that Mom will hardly notice! They are easy to make and can be stored in jars, or molded and put into a lipstick tube. Apply with a brush and remove with toner, flower water, or cleanser. You need half a quantity of the wax base made in Part 1 (below) for each color.

FIRST PINK

Makes 2–3 tubes or 10g jars

INGREDIENTS

PART 1

5 tsp castor oil

3g cosmetic beeswax

2g crushed carnauba wax

PART 2

Pigment colors/additions: ½ tsp pearl mica, ¼ tsp D&C red 27

3 drops vitamin E oil (optional)

2 drops strawberry aroma flavor or glycerin-based food flavoring (optional)

EQUIPMENT

Measuring spoons

Scales

Double boiler

Stirring spoon

Thermometer

Pestle and mortar

Small heat-resistant beaker with pouring lip

10g jars with screw cap or lipstick molds (see page 47) and tubes

PART 1

1 To make the wax base, put the ingredients into the upper pan of the double boiler and put hot water in the lower pan. Heat gently until the wax is just melted (do not exceed 160°F). Set aside.

BELOW If you are making your lipstick in a tube, measure the diameter of the tube to be sure that you lipstick fits the container.

From top to bottom: First Pink, Junior High, Pink Frost, and Cutesy Sparkle.

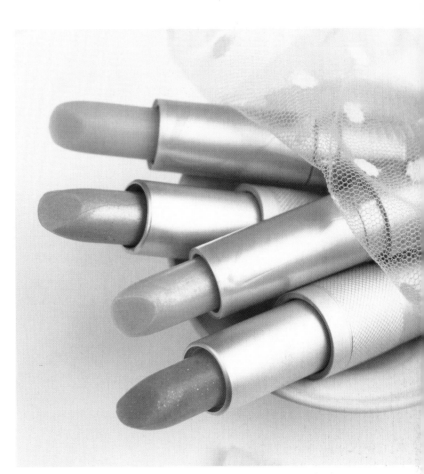

PART 2

2 Place all of the ingredients in a mortar. Mix well with the pestle, pressing out all of the lumps and air pockets. Transfer to a heat-resistant beaker.

3 Reheat the wax base (see Part 1, left) and quickly mix half of it with the Part 2 ingredients.

4 Fill jars to the base of the thread line or pour into your bought or homemade lipstick mold (see page 47). Pour the mixture carefully and protect your hands; the mixture is hot. Let it set for 1–2 hours and then insert into a lipstick tube.

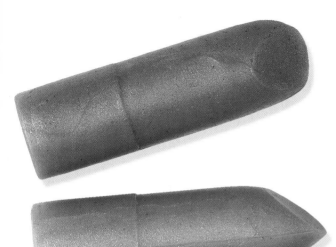

JUNIOR HIGH

Pigment colors/additions
½ tsp pearl mica
¼ tsp (F)D&C yellow 6 aluminum lake

PART 1
1 Follow the ingredients and instructions for Part 1 (see page 45).

PART 2
2 Follow the ingredients and instructions for Part 2 (see page 45), but use the colors/additions specified above.

Beauty tip
This is a peach-toned lip gloss with pearl to make your lips shine.

CUTESY SPARKLE

Pigment colors/additions
(+/-) ¼ tsp D&C red 30
Pinch of white crystallina frosting

PART 1
1 Follow the ingredients and instructions for Part 1 (see page 45).

PART 2
2 Follow the ingredients and instructions for Part 2 (see page 45), but use the colors/additions specified above.

Beauty tip
This transparent lip gloss has a hint of crystal sparkle. Apply over a deeper, matte color for extra glossiness.

ABOVE *These frosted, glossy tones moisturize your lips as well as giving them a hint of color.*

HOMEMADE LIPSTICK MOLD

If you can't get hold of a customized mold, it's really easy to make your own.

EQUIPMENT

2½in square of aluminum foil per mold
Pen or dowel with ¼in diameter (average size of a lipstick tube)
Ramekin or small dish filled with flour

I Wrap a foil square around the end of a pen or dowel; let a little of the foil overhang and twist to seal.

2 Gently push the wrapped pen or dowel – foil-sealed end first – into the flour-filled dish or ramekin. Carefully remove the dowel or pen; the foil tube should be standing upright.

3 Once you have prepared your lipstick mixture, carefully pour it into the foil tubes. Protect your hands as the mixture is hot. Reserve a little mixture for topping up.

4 Leave to set in a cool room for 1–2 hours. If any shrinkage occurs, reheat the reserved mixture and top up.

5 Once set, peel back the foil and insert into a lipstick tube. Carefully trim the exposed end to a "bullet" shape if you wish.

PINK FROST

Pigment colors/additions
¼ tsp pearl mica
¼ tsp mixed D&C red 21 and D&C red 30

PART 1
I Follow the ingredients and instructions for Part 1 (see page 45).

PART 2
2 Follow the ingredients and instructions for Part 2 (see page 45), but use the colors/additions specified above.

Beauty tip
A little more color pigment is added to this recipe for a sheer, pearlized lip tint.

BELOW *Before reusing lipstick tubes, remove all lipstick traces, and clean and sterilize thoroughly. Push-up or wind-up tubes are equally good.*

AUTUMN TINTS

Beautifully rich, strong shades to create dramatic full-lipped effects, particularly suited to darker skins. You need half a quantity of the wax base made in Part I (right) for each color.

RUSSET

Makes 2–3 tubes or 10g jars

INGREDIENTS

PART I

5 tsp castor oil

3g cosmetic beeswax

2g crushed carnauba wax

¼ tsp cocoa butter

¼ tsp glycerin

PART 2

Pigment colors/additions: ½ tsp pearl mica, ¼ tsp red iron oxide, ¼ tsp D&C red 7, pinch copper lip-grade glitter

3 drops vitamin E oil (optional)

EQUIPMENT

Measuring spoons

Scales

Double boiler

Stirring spoon

Thermometer

Pestle and mortar

Small heat-resistant beaker with pouring lip

10g jars with screw cap or lipstick molds (see page 47) and tubes

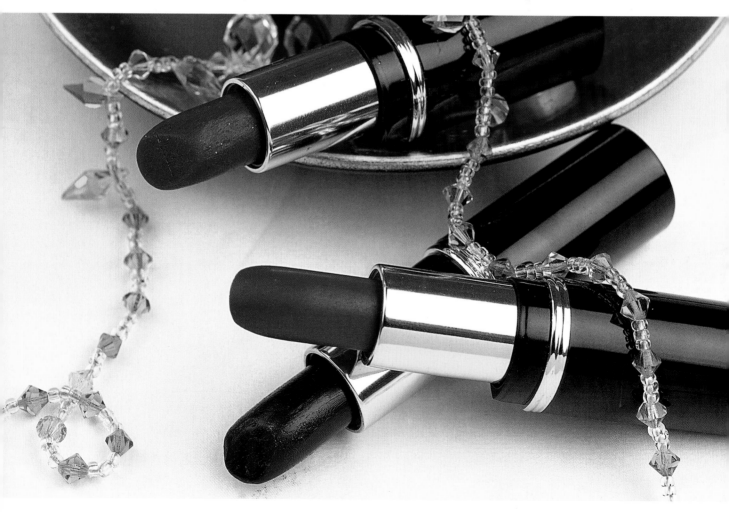

PART 1

1 To make the wax base, put the ingredients into the upper pan of the double boiler and put hot water into the lower pan. Heat gently until the wax is just melted (do not exceed 160°F). Set aside.

PART 2

2 Place all of the ingredients in a mortar. Mix well with the pestle, pressing out all of the lumps and air pockets. Transfer to a heat-resistant beaker.

3 Reheat the wax base (see Part 1, above) and quickly mix half of it with the Part 2 ingredients.

4 Fill jars to the base of thread line or pour into your bought or homemade lipstick molds (see page 47). Pour the mixture carefully and protect your hands as the mixture is hot. Let it set for 1–2 hours and then insert into a lipstick tube.

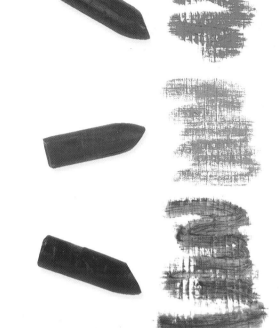

GOLDEN RED

Pigment colors/additions
½ tsp pearl mica
¼ tsp yellow iron oxide
¼ tsp red iron oxide
¼ tsp D&C red 7
Pinch gold lip-grade cosmetic glitter

PART 1

1 Follow the ingredients and instructions for Part 1 (above).

PART 2

2 Follow the ingredients and instructions for Part 2 (above), but use the pigment colors/additions specified above instead.

RUBY

Pigment colors/additions
¼ tsp D&C red 7
¼ tsp D&C red 34
¼ tsp D&C red 22

PART 1

1 Follow the ingredients and instructions for Part 1 (above left).

PART 2

2 Follow the ingredients and instructions for Part 2 (above left), but use the pigment colors/additions specified above instead.

Beauty tip
A rich-red color with a hint of gold is dramatic and sophisticated.

Beauty tip
The deep colors of red wine in a rich glossy lip color work for incredibly special occasions.

LEFT *If you use these rich colors on your lips, you should only use very light colors on your eyes.*

ABOVE RIGHT *From top to bottom: Ruby, Golden Red, and Russet.*

MOISTURIZING LIP COLORS

Lips can easily become dry, chapped, and damaged, due to harsh weather or lack of moisture. When the body is dehydrated, the mouth will develop a dry, crumpled appearance very quickly, so drinking lots of water helps maintain the beauty of your mouth. These moisturizing lipsticks will give good color and have beneficial properties. You need half a quantity of the wax base made in Part 1 (below) for each color.

SIXTIES PINK

Makes 2–3 tubes or 10g jars

INGREDIENTS
PART 1
5 tsp castor oil
3g cosmetic beeswax
3g crushed carnauba wax
1 tsp aloe vera gel
½ tsp calendula oil
2 drops benzoin resinoid essential oil

PART 2
Pigment colors/additions: ½ tsp pearl mica, ¼ tsp D&C red 21

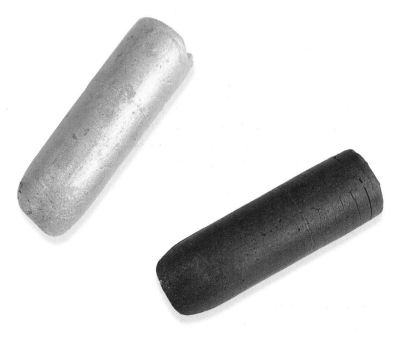

EQUIPMENT
Measuring spoons
Scales
Double boiler
Stirring spoon
Thermometer
Pestle and mortar
Small heat-resistant beaker with pouring lip
10g jars with screw cap or lipstick molds (see page 47) and tubes

PART 1
1 To make the wax base, put the ingredients into the upper pan of a double boiler and put hot water into the lower pan. Heat gently until the wax is just melted (do not exceed 160°F). Set aside.

PART 2
2 Place all of the ingredients in a mortar. Mix well with the pestle, pressing out all of the lumps and air pockets. Transfer to the heat-resistant beaker.
3 Reheat the wax base (see Part 1, above) and quickly mix half of it with the Part 2 ingredients.
4 Fill jars to the base of thread line or pour into your bought or homemade lipstick mold (see page 47). Pour the mixture carefully and protect your hands as the mixture is hot. Let it set for 1–2 hours and then insert into a lipstick tube.

BRONZE BERRY

Pigment colors/additions
¼ tsp brown iron oxide
¼ tsp red iron oxide
¼ tsp pearl mica or lip-grade gold or bronze glitter (optional)

PART 1
1 Follow the ingredients and instructions for Part 1 (see above).

PART 2
2 Follow the instructions for Part 2 (see above), but use the pigment colors/additions specified above instead.

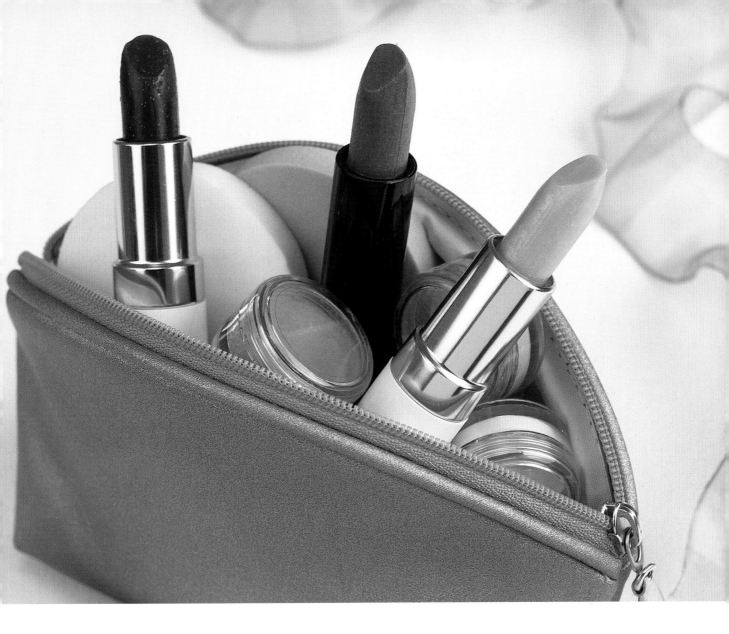

RED SHE SAID

Pigments colors/additions
¼ tsp D&C red 7
¼ tsp D&C red 22
To cool the tone: use few grains of D&C red 33 (too much and it will turn purple)
To warm the tone: use few grains of D&C red 6

PART I
I Follow the ingredients and instructions for Part I (see left).

PART 2
2 Follow the instructions for Part 2 (see left), but use the pigment colors/additions specified above instead.

Tip
Achieving a true, attractive red color for a lipstick takes practice. Generally, carmine is used for pigments with blue or yellow tones, but carmine is made from the cochineal insect, and I prefer not to use it.

ABOVE *From left to right: Bronze Berry, Red She Said, and Sixties Pink.*

SPLATTER COLORS

These colors are great fun to make and wear. You can use the technique described below with any of the lipstick mixtures and colors in this chapter and also the Frosted Shadows for your eyes (see pages 28–34). You need to work quickly, and the effects are never the same twice. When you pour the colors, the jar needs to be on the move – I use a children's spinning painting wheel, but a pottery wheel or even an old record player (set on high speed) will work. I would recommend that you use a microwave to reheat your mixtures since you may need to do this several times. Reheating the mixture for approximately 10 seconds should keep the waxes liquid.

INGREDIENTS

See the relevant recipes for the 2–3 colors that you
  have chosen.

EQUIPMENT

(See the relevant recipes that you have chosen, plus
items listed below)
Reusable adhesive pads
Jars with sides at least 3in high
Turntable (painting or pottery wheel, old record player)
Heat-resistant glass or plastic beaker with pouring lip
Protective eye goggles

1 Make the two or three different colors that you
  have chosen.
2 Place an adhesive pad on the base of the jar and stick it
  to the turntable.
3 Keeping the turntable still, pour a fine layer of the first
  color into the jar. Let it set for 2 minutes.
4 Put on the protective eye goggles. Spin the turntable
  quickly and carefully pour in a stream of the second
  color. The speed will splatter this color over the first
  layer. Switch off the turntable and let the mixture cool.
5 Add the third color as before, slightly altering the
  pouring angle to give a different pattern.
6 You can repeat this method as required.

RIGHT *The great thing about using your Splatter Colors is that you will get a different effect every time you use them.*

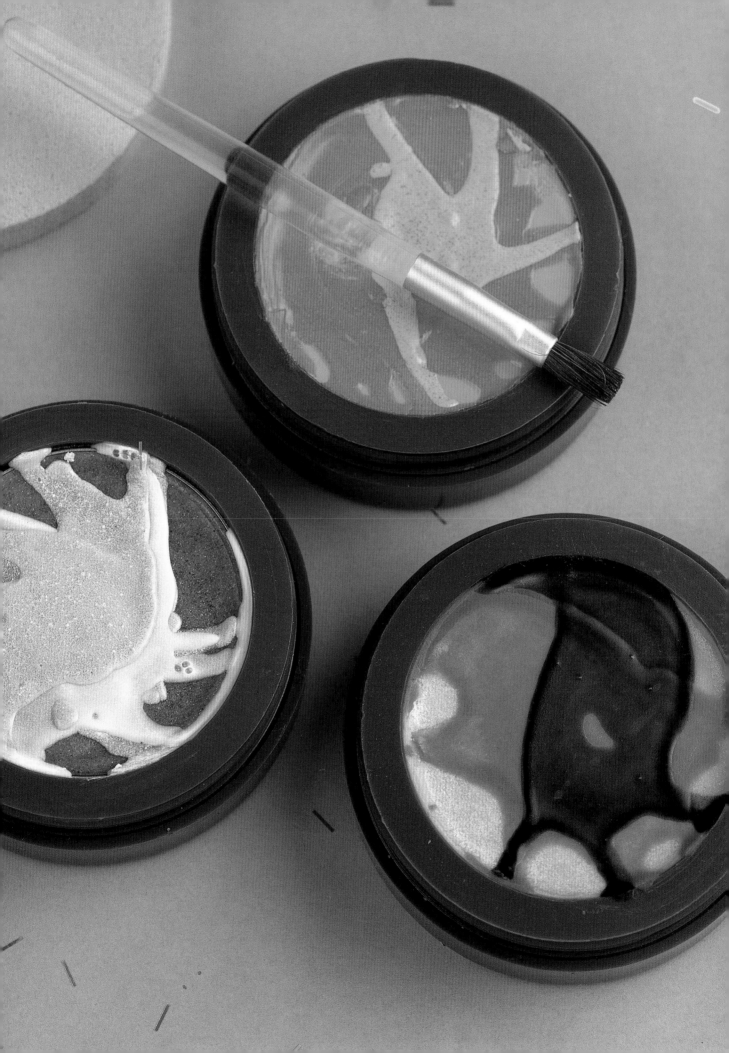

LIPS TO SHOCK!

Bright and amusing colors can be made using strong, single tones. They are great for parties and dressing up. You need half a quantity of the wax base made in Part 1 (below) for each color.

ELECTRIC BLUE

Makes 2–3 x 10g jars

INGREDIENTS
PART 1
5 tsp castor oil
3g cosmetic beeswax
2g crushed carnauba wax
2g shea butter

PART 2
Pigment colors/additions: ½ tsp (F)D&C blue no.1 aluminum lake, pinch (external use) black iron oxide

EQUIPMENT
Measuring spoons
Scales
Double boiler
Stirring spoon
Thermometer
Pestle and mortar
Small heat-resistant beaker with pouring lip
10g jars with screw-caps

PART 1
1 To make the wax base, put the ingredients into the upper pan of the double boiler and put hot water in the lower pan. Heat gently until the wax is melted (do not exceed 160°F). Set aside.

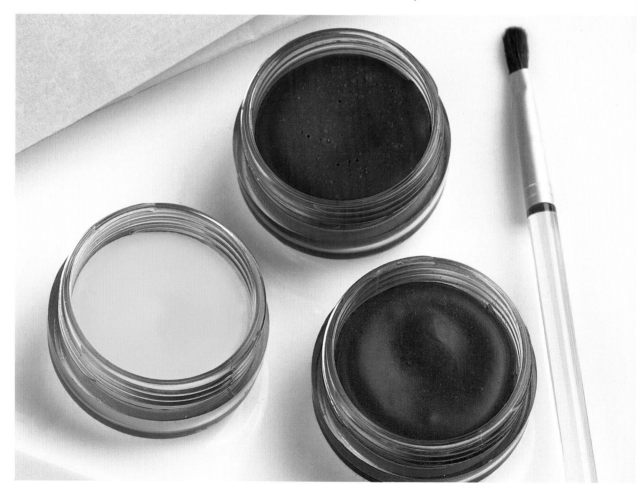

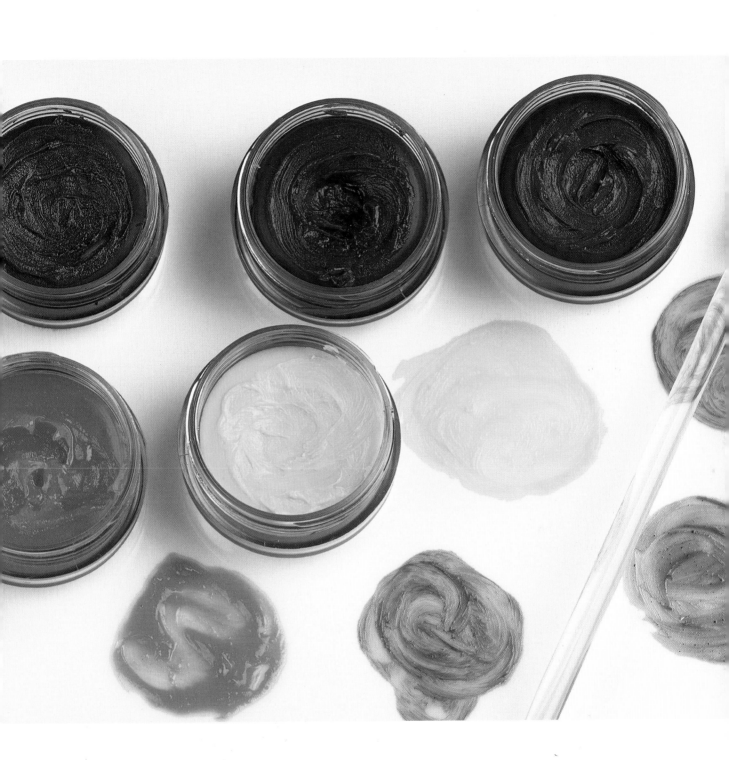

PART 2

2 Place all of the ingredients in a mortar. Mix well with the pestle, pressing out all of the lumps and air pockets. Transfer to the heat-resistant beaker.

3 Reheat the wax base (see Part 1, above left) and quickly mix half of it with the Part 2 ingredients.

4 Fill jars to the base of thread line and set for 1–2 hours.

LEFT *Dry lips can absorb lip shades. Apply an undercoat of sheer color or lip balm if your lips are prone to absorbing lip colors.*

ABOVE *London and Paris have many shops selling wild lipstick colors. These are copies of some of the more unusual shades that I have seen.*

GHOULISH GREEN

Pigment colors/additions
¼ tsp pearl mica
½ tsp (F)D&C yellow no. 5 aluminum lake
¼ tsp (F)D&C blue no. 1 aluminum lake
Tiny pinch (external use) black iron oxide

PART 1
1 Follow the ingredients and instructions for Part 1 (see page 54).

PART 2
2 Follow the instructions for Part 2 (see page 55), but use the pigment colors/additions specified above instead.

PASSIONATE IN PURPLE

Pigment colors/additions
¼ tsp D&C red 33
¼ tsp D&C red 7

PART 1
1 Follow the ingredients and instructions for Part 1 (see page 54).

PART 2
2 Follow the instructions for Part 2 (see page 55), but use the pigment colors/additions specified above instead.

LASER ORANGE

Pigment colors/additions
¼ tsp (F)D&C yellow no. 6 aluminum lake
¼ tsp pearl mica
Pinch gold cosmetic-grade glitter (must be suitable for use in lipsticks)

PART 1
1 Follow the instructions for Part 1 (see page 54).

PART 2
2 Follow the instructions for Part 2 (see page 55), but use the pigment colors/additions specified above instead. Add the glitter just before pouring the mixture into the jars.

GOLDEN YELLOW

Pigment colors/additions
¼ tsp (F)D&C yellow no. 5 aluminum lake
¼ tsp pearl mica
Pinch gold cosmetic-grade glitter (must be suitable for use in lipsticks)

PART 1
1 Follow the ingredients and instructions for Part 1 (see page 54).

PART 2
2 Follow the instructions for Part 2 (see page 55), but use the pigment colors/additions specified above instead. Add the glitter just before pouring the mixture into the jars.

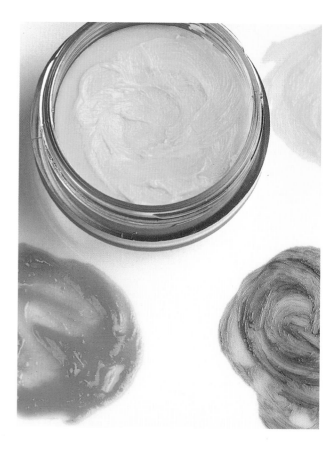

ABOVE *Golden yellow lips look fantastic with sparkling colors on the eyes and dark mascara.*

LIP BALM

Lip balms or ointments are moisturizing, hydrating, and protective. They can heal lips that are dry, cracked, and in need of tender loving care. You may choose any combination of essential oils and fragrances (see page 83), but keep the dilution very low; alternatively use the essential oils suggested below.

Makes 2–3 x 20g jars

INGREDIENTS

1 tbsp sweet almond oil
10g cocoa butter
2 tsp calendula oil
5g cosmetic beeswax
6 drops benzoin resinoid oil
4 drops lavender essential oil
4 drops geranium essential oil

EQUIPMENT

Double boiler
Measuring spoons
Scales
Stirring spoon
Jars

1 Put hot water in the lower pan of the double boiler. Put the sweet almond oil, cocoa butter, and calendula oil in the upper pan and heat gently.

2 Add the beeswax and let it melt.

3 Add the benzoin resinoid oil to the mix and stir well.

4 Remove from the heat. Add the essential oils to the mix and quickly pour into jars. Reserve approximately 2 tablespoonfuls.

5 Let the mixture cool. If a well appears in the finished product, it can be filled with the reserved mix (you can reheat the mix as necessary).

RIGHT *The natural ingredients in this lip balm will remain active for 6–12 months. Store in a cool place.*

QUICK LIP BALM

In a double boiler, heat 50ml sweet almond oil and 6g beeswax until the wax melts. Add 1–2 drops of food or aroma flavor such as vanilla or peppermint. Pour into jars and leave to set.

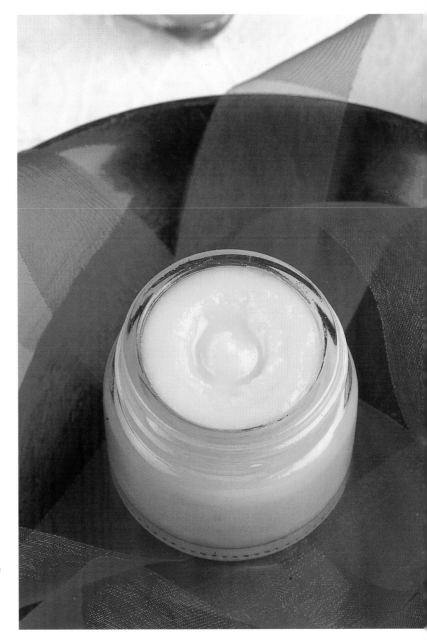

FACE BASE

By using foundation and concealers, blemishes and imperfections can be disguised. The recipes in this chapter are suitable for many skin tones. The concealer contains natural essential oils to make a healing, soothing stick unlike anything else available. There is a selection suitable for all skin types and for makeup users of different ages. I have included some tips on successful application to help your skin look natural. All of the products can be applied with a sponge, pad, or brush.

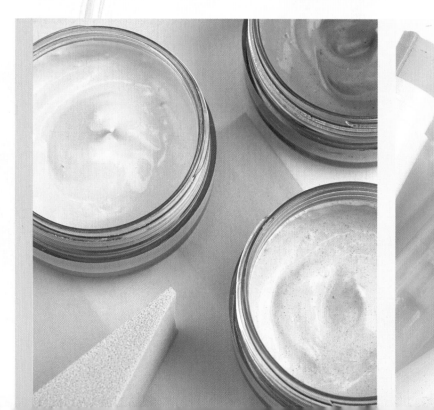

FOUNDATION

Foundation is a tinted layer of makeup worn directly on the face, neck, and décolleté. It creates a subtle layer of color to give a "blank canvas" on which to build color. It can add lift and light and improve the appearance of the complexion. Foundations can be lightly tinted moisturizers or rich color creams, and have matte or silk-effect finishes. Some foundations are medicated, containing antibacterial agents.

A foundation needs to match your natural skin tone. Once you have mixed your color, it's a good idea to mix two other variations of this tone – one for the summer, when your skin is slightly darker, and one for the winter, when it is lighter. Skin tones are a combination of brown, yellow, and red. The main pigment colors to build these are red, pink, black, brown, and yellow, plus green, white, and blue. Fortunately, iron oxides (particularly the browns) cover many shade variations and mix well with red and yellow iron oxides. Start with brown shades, add yellow, then modify with red and white. Blue and green take away redness; black and blue darken tones.

TINTED CREAM FOUNDATION

These foundations should be applied with a damp sponge and removed with cleanser. This is the basic recipe with specific color blends listed on page 62.

Makes 100–125g of product

INGREDIENTS
PART 1
1 tsp magnesium stearate
1 tsp kaolin
½ tsp talcum
½ tsp cornstarch
¼ tsp potato starch
Chosen colors (see page 62)

PART 2
65ml purified water
1 tsp glycerin
2 drops germaben II

PART 3
½ tsp cetyl alcohol
2g cosmetic beeswax
5g shea butter
15g jojoba oil

PART 4
2–3 drops tea tree essential oil
2–3 drops lavender essential oil

EQUIPMENT
Measuring spoons
Bowls
Stirring spoon
Pestle and mortar
Measuring cup
Scales
Small stainless steel saucepan
Double boiler
Thermometer
Balloon whisk
Screw-cap jar

PART 1

1 Mix the powders in a bowl. Place 1 teaspoon of the mixed powder in a mortar. Add your chosen colors. Mix well to blend color thoroughly. Set aside.

PART 2

2 Heat the purified water in a stainless steel pan, over very gentle heat, to boiling point. Add the glycerin and germaben II. Let it cool while you make Part 3 (below).

PART 3

3 Place all the ingredients in the upper pan of the double boiler and put hot water in the lower pan. Heat gently until just melted (do not exceed 160°F).

4 Add the reserved Part 2 mixture and blend together. If they separate, simply reheat. Use a balloon whisk and start to form an emulsion.

5 Set aside 1 teaspoon of Part 1 for color adjustments if required and then gradually fold the remaining powder into the emulsion until it is thoroughly incorporated.

PART 4

6 Add the essential oils, stirring carefully. Whisk gently to blend the ingredients uniformly. If the mixture is a little pale, add a matchhead of the reserved Part 1 powder to adjust the depth of color.

7 Pour into a screw-cap jar. Store in a cool place. Use within 4 weeks.

BELOW *Creamy, moisturizing, and sheer – this recipe is suitable for young or combination skin because it will never look caked or heavy.*

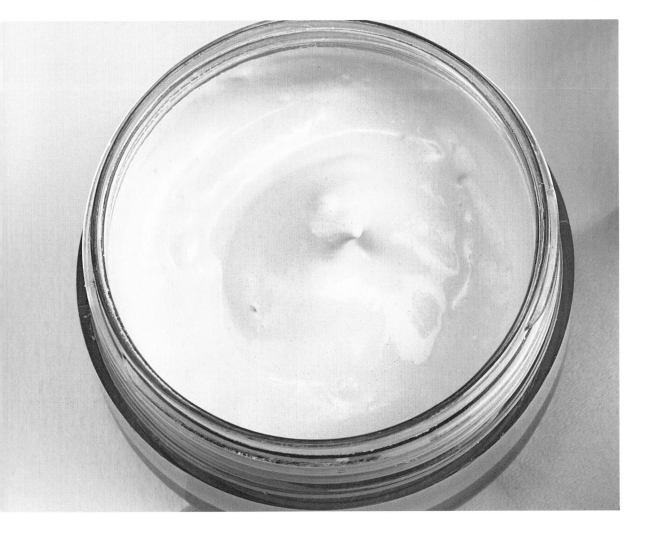

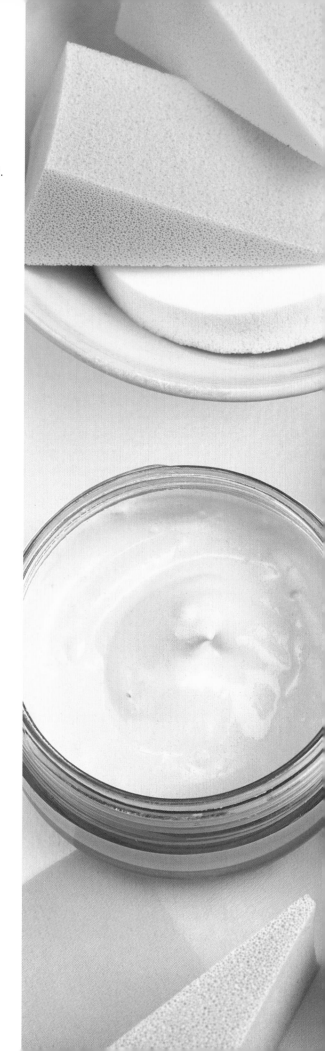

The following color blends should be added with Part I (see page 60). The names of the recipes refer to skin tone rather than the color of the mixture. Mix the powders in a mortar, using a pestle, and add as directed.

PEACHES AND CREAM
¼ tsp red/yellow blend iron oxide (CI 77491/2)
Pinch brown made up of red/yellow/black iron oxides
Few grains red and/or yellow iron oxide
Blend and adjust with titanium dioxide to make a total
 of ½ tsp color

OLIVE
¼ tsp brown made up of red/yellow/black iron oxides
 (CI 77491 mahogany tone)
⅛ tsp yellow iron oxide
Few grains red iron oxide
Few grains chromium oxide green
Blend and adjust with titanium dioxide to make a total
 of ½ tsp color

DARK
½ tsp brown made up of red/yellow/black/nut brown
 iron oxides (CI 77491/2/9)
Few grains (external use) black iron oxide
Few grains ultramarine blue
Few grains yellow and/or red iron oxide
Blend and adjust with titanium dioxide to make a total
 of ½ tsp color

IVORY PALE
Few grains each brown iron oxide mix
Yellow iron oxide
Few grains ultramarine blue
¼ tsp titanium dioxide
½ tsp white kaolin to disperse

BRONZING
¼ tsp red iron oxide base
¼ tsp pearl mica (gold if available)
Few grains yellow iron oxide
½ tsp talcum to disperse
Pinch fine gold cosmetic-grade glitter (optional)

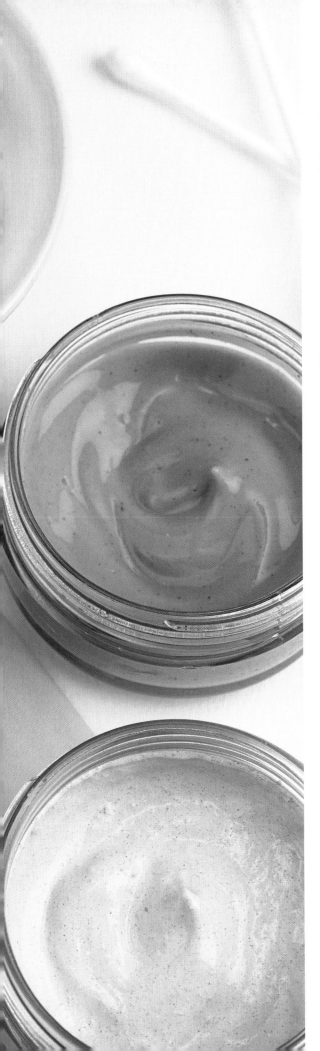

Tips

You can adjust any of the recipes to create just the right color for you. You may find minute quantities of D&C red 7 calcium lake, and D&C orange 4 particularly useful. These colors have a natural quality and create a balancing, translucent color.

Adjust your color base with titanium dioxide when your complexion is paler i.e. in winter, and with brown, blue, and black pigment colors when it is darker.

Making a concentrated base of your favorite color combination can be useful when repeating your recipe or altering the tone according to seasons. Pigment colors may be dry-mixed and kept in a sealed jar for up to 18 months.

LEFT *Peaches and Cream (left), Dark (top right), and Olive (bottom right). Once you are used to handling the color pigments, you can adjust the recipes shown on these pages to better suit your skin tone.*

LOOSE POWDER FOUNDATION

Makes 50g of product

Use the same color mixes for this loose powder as for the cream foundations. If you don't add any color pigments, you have a translucent powder. Use sparingly; otherwise, you may look too pale. Apply with a dry powder puff, large brush, or sponge.

INGREDIENTS

PART 1
½ tsp magnesium stearate
1 tsp kaolin
1 tsp talcum
½ tsp cornstarch
Pinch potato starch

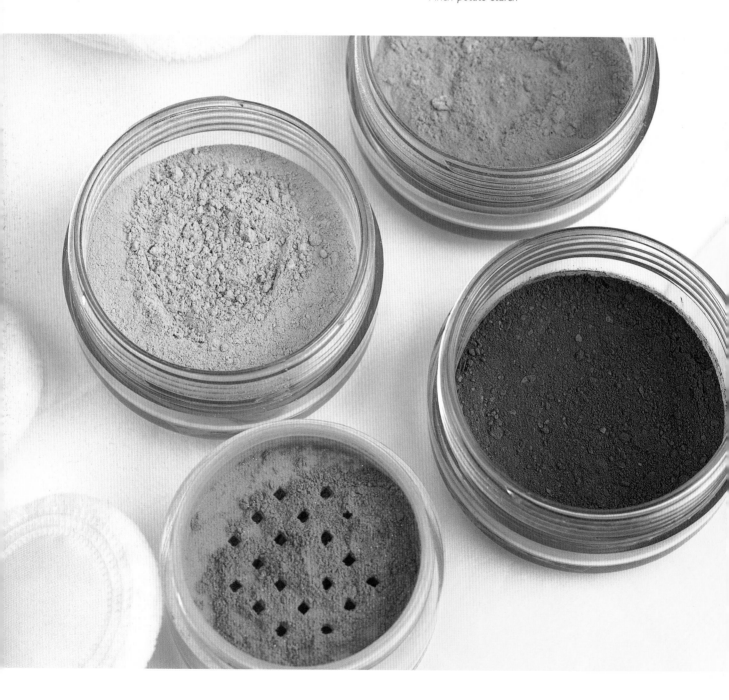

PART 2

tsp jojoba oil

—4 drops of jojoba to mix

drops tea tree and/or 2 drops lavender essential oil (optional)

PART 3

tsp of chosen mixed color pigments (see page 62)

titanium dioxide

EQUIPMENT

Measuring spoons

Pestle and mortar

Stirring spoon

Sifter jars

PART 1

1 Mix the powders in a mortar using the pestle. Reserve 1 teaspoonful.

PART 2

2 Add the teaspoon of jojoba oil to Part 1 and mix with the pestle until fully absorbed.

3 Add the essential oils and blend thoroughly.

PART 3

4 Carefully incorporate the mixed color powder into the mixture a little at a time. Stop when you've added enough color. If required, adjust color with titanium dioxide. Pulverize with the pestle for at least 3 minutes to make sure that the ingredients are well blended.

5 Put into jars.

LEFT *Peaches and Cream (left), Bronzing (top), and Dark (right) foundations work well with a brown or ruby blusher (bottom).*

RIGHT *These powder foundations are great to make, as you literally watch the color develop before your eyes. Don't be tempted to add more color; mix the quantity specified for 2–3 minutes and watch the magic.*

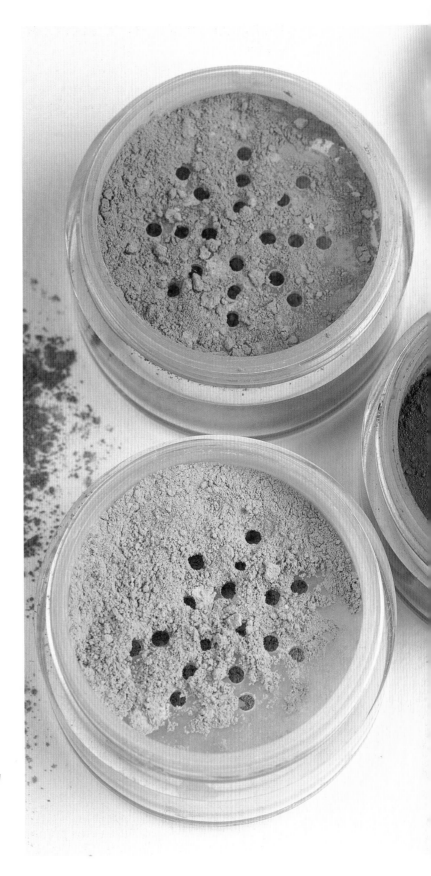

CREAM CONCEALER

Concealer improves the appearance of blemished skin and hides dark circles under the eyes and broken veins across the nose and cheeks. Store in a jar or put the stick into a lip balm or push-up tube dispenser. Using the stick straight on the skin may spread infection if used on spots and pimples, so apply with a sponge or brush and wash it after each use. Remove with cleanser and an astringent toner. You need half a quantity of wax base for each color.

Makes 2 tubes or a 15g jar

INGREDIENTS

PART 1
1 tbsp jojoba oil
½ tsp cosmetic beeswax
½ tsp crushed carnauba wax
Pinch stearic acid flakes
2 drops tea tree and/or lavender essential oil

PART 2
¼ tsp mixed pigment color powders (see page 62; use a slightly
*   paler shade than your normal skin tone)*
Few grains ultramarine blue
¼ tsp talcum
⅛ tsp cornstarch
3g titanium dioxide

EQUIPMENT
Measuring spoons
Double boiler
Stirring spoon
Thermometer
Scales
Pestle and mortar
Small heat-resistant beaker with pouring lip
Jars or push-up tube dispensers

LEFT *Choose concealers one or two shades lighter than your skin tone to help reduce the appearance of dark circles and conceal blemishes.*

RIGHT *These tubes make great containers for concealers, lipsticks, and balms. There is no need to mold before use, just fill the container and let it set.*

PART 1
1 Put the ingredients into the upper pan of the double boiler. Fill the lower pan with hot water. Heat gently until the wax melts (do not exceed 160°F). Set aside.

PART 2
2 Mix all of the ingredients in a mortar using the pestle. Mix well, pressing out all of the lumps and air pockets. Transfer to the flameproof beaker.
3 Reheat half of the Part 1 wax mixture and quickly mix with Part 2.
4 Carefully pour the hot mixture into jars or tubes. Protect your hands as the wax mixture is hot! Reserve a little mixture for topping up.
5 Leave to set for 1-2 hours in a cool room. There may be a little shrinkage. Just reheat the reserved mixture and and top up.

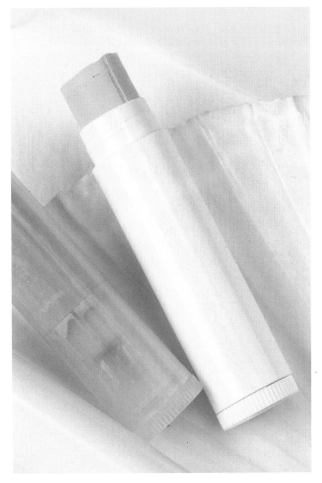

BLUSH POWDER

Blush powder is a darkened brown or red tone powder makeup used to accentuate the cheekbones. It can also appear to alter the shape of the face by creating shadow, or giving the impression of shade. For example, shading a round face with a darker tone on the jaw line will elongate the face. Blush powder gives "color" to the skin and may improve a bland complexion. We now use subtle shades and frosting, yet historically blusher has been, at extremes, bright red spots of color on the cheeks. Rosy cheeks were said to be a sign of health and long life. Apply blusher over foundation with a large powder brush (always shake away excess before applying) as the last and finishing color. You could also apply with a dry powder puff or sponge. Remove with a suitable cleanser.

LEFT *This brush is just the right size (1 in in diameter) for applying blusher. If you use a larger brush, the blusher tends to color too large an area of the cheek.*

Makes 50g of product

INGREDIENTS

PART 1

½ tsp magnesium stearate
1 tsp kaolin
1 tsp talcum
½ tsp cornstarch

PART 2

1 tsp jojoba oil
2–4 drops of jojoba oil to mix

PART 3

½ tsp of blended blusher powder pigment (see color mixes opposite)

EQUIPMENT

Measuring spoons
Pestle and mortar
Sifter jars

PART 1

1 Mix the powders in a mortar using a pestle. Set aside 1 teaspoonful for any color adjustments.

PART 2

2 Add 1 teaspoonful of jojoba oil, drop by drop to the Part 1 powders. Mix with the pestle until the oil is absorbed.

PART 3

3 Carefully incorporate the blended pigment powders a little at a time. Stop when enough color has been added. Adjust with titanium dioxide if required. Pulverize in the mortar, using the pestle for at least 3 minutes to prevent streaks when the makeup is applied to the skin. Add a drop or two of jojoba oil if the mix is very dusty.

4 Store in a sifter jar.

Beauty tip

If you are applying shading color, the color should be applied in a slight curve along the lower side of the cheekbone.

The following color blends make up Part 3 (opposite). Simply mix the powders in a mortar, using a pestle, and add as directed.

PINK AND RUBY

¼ tsp brown iron oxide
Few grains D&C red 7
Few grains red iron oxide
Adjust with titanium dioxide (up to ¼ tsp)

BROWN AND BRONZE

¼ tsp basic brown iron oxide base
⅛ tsp yellow iron oxide
Few grains D&C red 6
Adjust with titanium dioxide (up to ¼ tsp)

COOLING SHADES

(+/-) ¼ tsp brown iron oxide base, yellow tone
Few grains chromium oxide green
Few grains yellow and red iron oxide, mix well for 2-3 minutes
Adjust with titanium dioxide (up to ⅛ tsp)

VAMP EFFECT

¼ tsp pearl mica
Few grains ultramarine violet CI 77007
Few grains red and yellow iron oxide, mix well for 2-3 minutes
¼ tsp talcum
¼ tsp kaolin

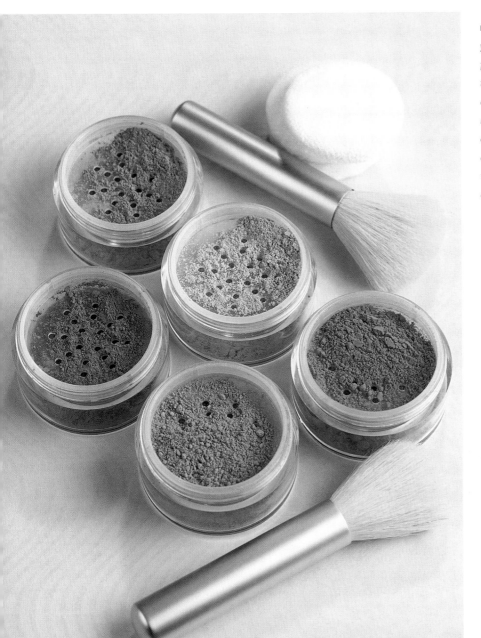

LEFT *You need to decide why you are applying blusher to your face. Are you trying to enhance the shape of your face or to add color? Both are valid reasons, but will affect your choice of color. Try out a few colors and adjust the recipes in this chapter to suit your skin color and face shape.*

PARTY TIME

Parties can be fun and wild, or sophisticated and businesslike. Sometimes they are a mixture of all of these things. Young fun means dressing up, being different, and giving life a sparkle, especially after exams, the end of a year, or the close of a stressful project. Party makeup is all about throwing caution to the wind and using color and sparkle. The recipes include an unusual array of body and hair cosmetics. Only make small quantities and above all, enjoy the party!

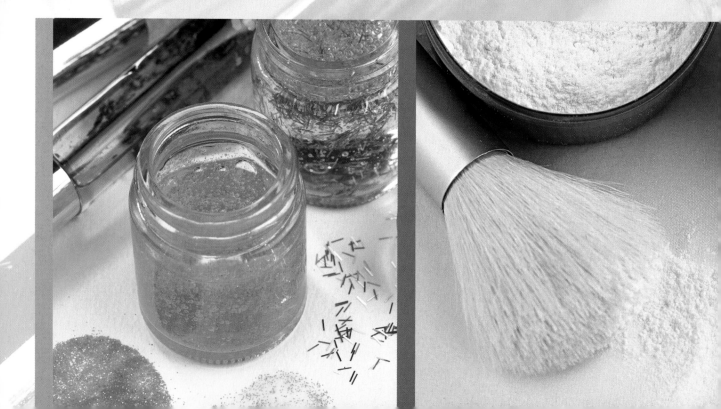

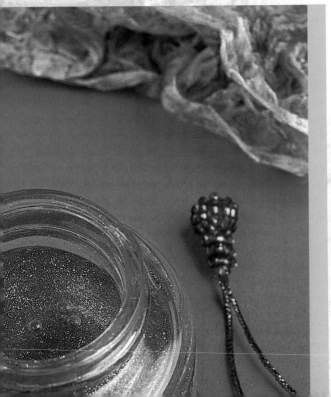

HAIR AND BODY GEL

Create fun effects with this hair and body gel. You must be sure to use colorfast cosmetic-grade glitter. Wash out of the hair with your normal shampoo or shower it off your body. This gel should not be used on the eyes.

Makes 100g of product

INGREDIENTS

PART 1

100ml aloe vera juice

2g guar or xanthan gum

6 drops germaben II or 6 drops paraben solution or 2g
  potassium sorbate (preservatives)

PART 2

½–1 tsp cosmetic-grade glitter (for example, flowers, hearts, gold
  stars, holographic laser shaves, silver glitter, crystallina)

Tip

It is not necessary to add a preservative to the gel unless you
plan to store it for more than two days.

EQUIPMENT

Measuring jug	*Kitchen scales*
Double boiler	*Stirring spoon*
Thermometer	*Measuring spoons*
	Clear, glass, screw-cap jars

PART 1

1 Put the aloe vera juice into the upper pan of the double boiler and hot water into the lower pan. Heat to 175°F. Remove from the heat.

2 Sprinkle the gum into the juice and mix quickly while it thickens. Add preservative and stir. Let it cool. This is the gel base.

PART 2

3 Add chosen glitter, stirring to suspend in gel. Put into jars. Shake before use.

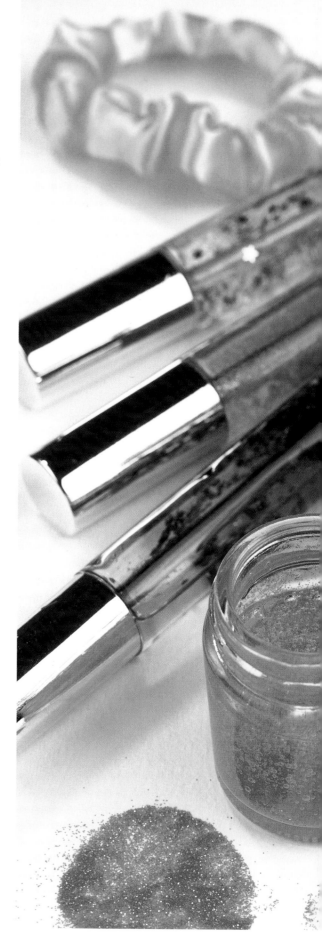

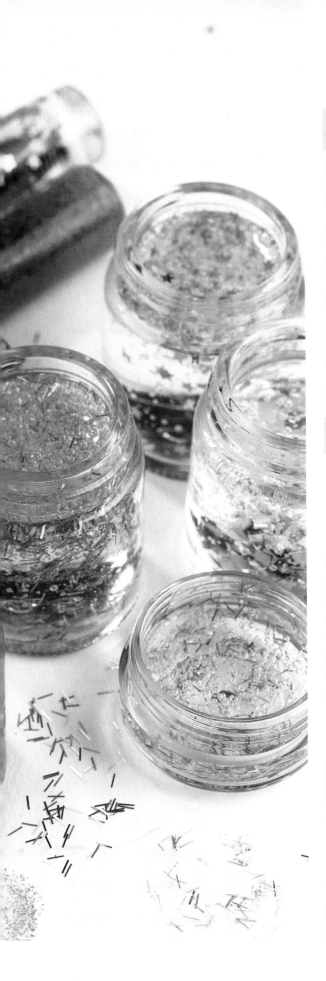

TO FILL A MASCARA TUBE

If you want to apply the gel to your hair, put the gel into a mascara tube.

1 Place a doughnut or cream attachment on an icing bag. Fill the bag with the glitter gel.
2 Remove the reducer from the tube because it may stop the gel from being applied to the brush and remove the glitter particles. Insert the nozzle into the tube and apply gentle pressure to the bag. Fill the tube.
3 Apply the gel to the hair by brushing the gel along the hair shaft – root to tip. The gel dries in 2–5 minutes. It may be set with non-aerosol hairspray if desired.

LEFT *Cosmetic-grade glitter is made without sharp edges. Stars and shapes may be used as a detail near the eyebrow or on the cheeks. Apply a few shapes, leave it to dry, and they should remain on the skin for a few hours.*

QUICK GLITTER GEL

Use ready-made, clear aloe vera gel (available in health food stores) and simply add cosmetic-grade glitter particles.

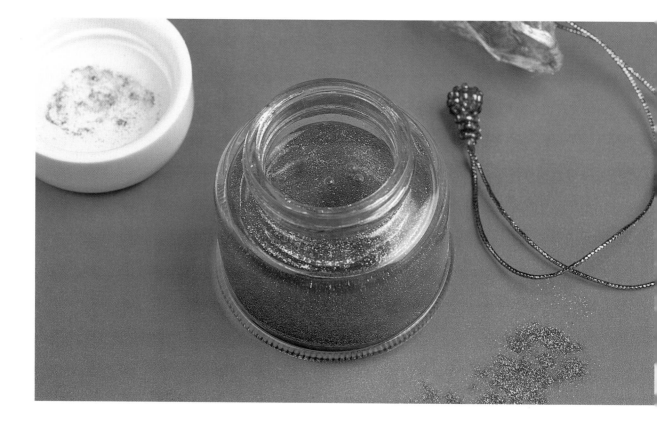

MIDAS TOUCH BODY GLITTER

Apply to your shoulders, arms, cheekbones – any area that needs sparkle! Shower off with your normal shower gel.

Makes 100g of product

INGREDIENTS
1 quantity gel base (Part 1, page 72)
1 tsp gold cosmetic-grade glitter

EQUIPMENT
Measuring cup/measuring spoons
Double boiler
Thermometer
Scales
Stirring spoon
Clear glass jars

1 Make the gel base (see Part 1, page 72).
2 Mix the gold glitter into the gel and blend thoroughly.
3 Put into small glass jars.

SPARKLING BODY DUST

A dusting talc to give sparkle to the skin. Fill talc shakers and shake onto your shoulders and arms.

Makes 20g of product

INGREDIENTS
1 tbsp talcum
1 tsp mica (pearl, gold, or colored)
½ tsp fine cosmetic crystallina
1 drop essential oil of your choice

EQUIPMENT
Measuring spoons
Medium plastic bag or screw-cap jar
Pestle and mortar
Talcum shaker

1 Put the powders into a bag or screw-cap jar. Shake to mix. Transfer to a mortar. Add the essential oil.
2 Incorporate using the pestle. Fill your shaker.

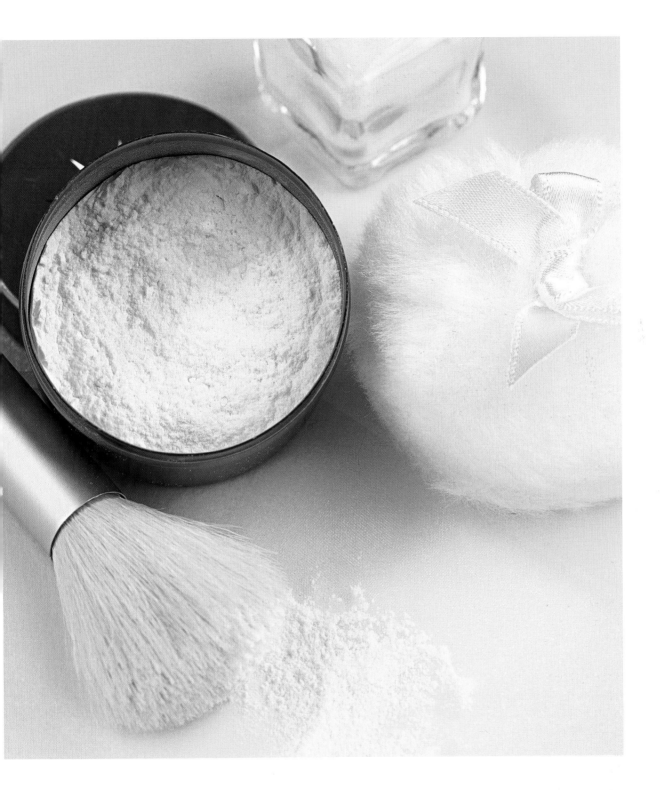

ABOVE LEFT *Fine gold cosmetic glitter adds a wonderful shimmer to the skin. Apply the glitter after dressing.*

ABOVE *Body dust will make your skin glisten. Vary the shades of mica to add a pearl shimmer on hot summer evenings.*

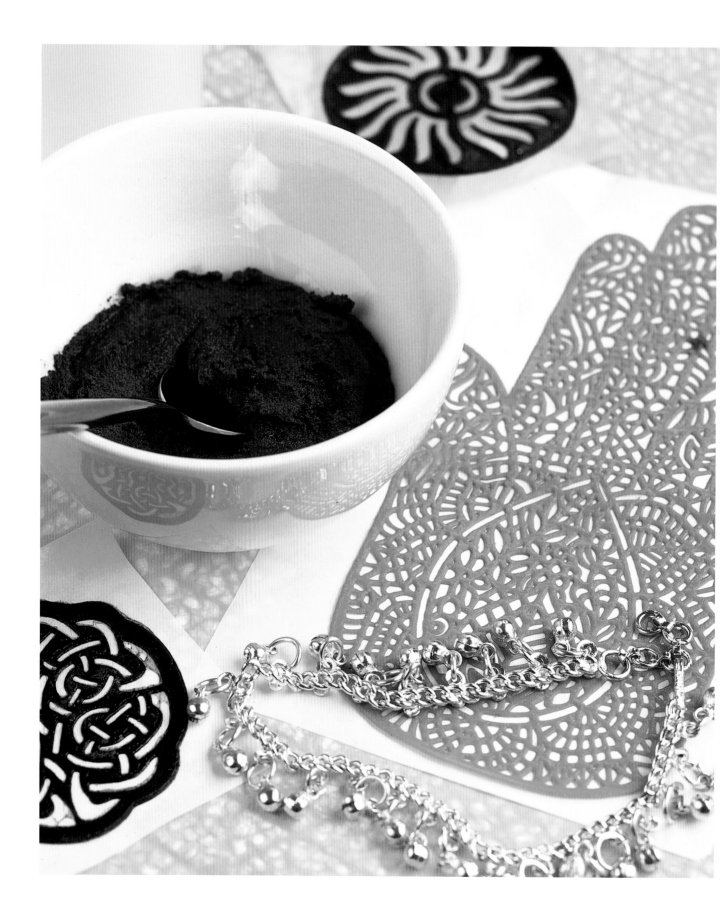

TEMPORARY HENNA TATTOO

Body decoration has always been popular. Historically, henna designs were used at bridal festivals to adorn the body, face, hands, and feet. The time the decoration remains on the skin varies from person to person; there will also be variations in color due to the acid balance of your skin and the environment. The more patience you have in allowing the color paste to develop, the better the results. Avoid touching the paste with your hands as you may stain your fingers, and make the fixative before you paint the tattoo.

Enough for 5 designs (depending on size)

INGREDIENTS
PART 1
HENNA PASTE

4 tbsp fresh lemon juice
10 drops clove oil
5 drops eucalyptus oil
2 tsp sugar
28g fresh green henna powder, sifted
½ tsp olive oil

PART 2
FIXATIVE

1 tbsp lemon juice
1½ tsp sugar
1 drop clove oil
1 drop eucalyptus oil

EQUIPMENT

Newspapers (to protect work area)
Juice squeezer
Pan
Thermometer
Measuring spoons
Heat-resistant bowl
Stirring spoon
Latex gloves
Scales
Sieve
Voile fabric or nylon hose
Small plastic bag
Plastic squeeze bottle with fine nozzle
Cotton pads

PART 1

1 Lay newspaper over your work area to protect it from becoming stained.
2 Warm the lemon juice in a pan to 140°F. Set aside.
3 Put the clove oil, eucalyptus oil, and sugar into a bowl. Stir until dissolved.
4 Wearing latex gloves, add the henna powder, half of the lemon juice, and the olive oil. Mix to a soft paste (like toothpaste), adding more lemon juice as necessary. If the mixture is lumpy, strain it through a piece of voile or nylon hose.
5 Place the mixture in a small, strong, but flexible plastic bag. Gather up the bag and seal the top (so that it resembles an icing bag) and snip off the corner. Carefully squeeze the mixture out of the bag into the bottle. Let it cure for 12-24 hours before use.

PART 2

6 Put the lemon juice and sugar in a pan. Heat gently until the sugar is dissolved. Remove from the heat and pour into a bowl.
7 Add the essential oils and mix well.
8 Paint the henna design. Once the painted design is starting to become matte (but not cracking), use a cotton pad to gently dab the fixative onto the design. Reapplying the fixative will prolong the henna design. It can be stored in the refrigerator for 28 days.

NOTE

Always use green henna, not the black variety, which has been shown to stain and damage skin. Avoid getting any henna on your nails. The nails absorb henna, and it will be almost impossible to remove the orange and brown stains. Washing any spilled paste off the skin near the decoration may damage the design due to water treatment chemicals.

LEFT *Intricate stencils made in traditional or contemporary designs make the application of henna paste even easier. Put the stencil on dry skin. Carefully cover with paste, allowing each space to fill wth henna mixture. Let it set for 10 minutes, then remove the stencil. Apply fixative.*

SKIN PREPARATION

If you are writing a letter, painting a picture, or preparing a meal, you start with a clean surface. The same principle applies to your skin. It must be cleaned and prepared before it is decorated with makeup. There are three stages – cleansing, toning, and moisturizing. Cleansing gives your skin a chance to find its natural balance, toning refreshes the skin, and the application of moisturizer is like feeding the skin.

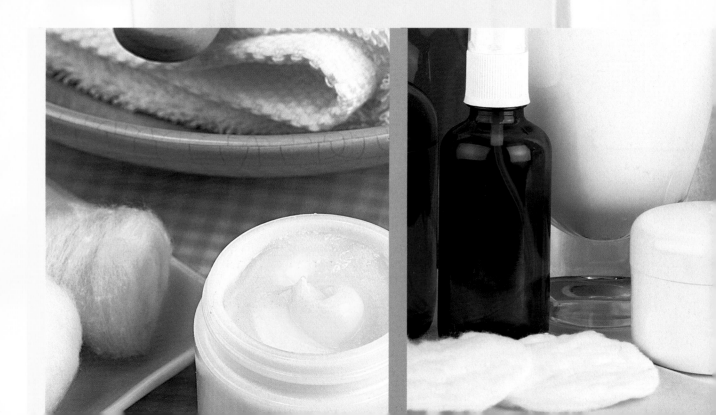

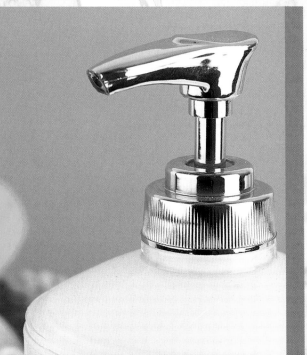

CLEANSING

The skin has many unseen enemies lying on its surface which need removing or cleansing to enable your skin to breathe and appear fresh.

There are five main contaminants that stick to the outer layer of the skin and require removal:

1 Loose skin cells that have not yet fallen from the skin.
2 Dust from the air around us.
3 Soot from fine particles of carbon in the air.
4 Salts and other secretions from the skin, such as urea. (If you have eaten foods that are unusual in your normal diet, such as strong garlic or spices, the aroma will be secreted onto the skin's surface.)
5 Bacteria, some of which naturally live on the skin, some from the atmosphere.

If you are wearing makeup, it also needs to be removed. Make-up is designed to adhere to the outer layer of skin. Therefore, the makeup needs to be removed with cleanser, and then you need to repeat the process to actually cleanse the skin itself. This is called double cleansing.

DOUBLE CLEANSING

Cleansing the skin of the build up of contaminants and makeup involves using removers. These can be in the form of soaps, gels, or cleansing lotions. Commercial soap is generally thought of as being unsuitable for your face, but a little powdered, natural handmade soap in your cleanser will not dry or damage the skin; however, you should not use it around the delicate eye areas.

The impurities can also be dissolved by using an oil-based product, such as cleansing creams, cold creams, or vegetable oils to "float" the impurities from the skin. If you live in a heavily built-up traffic zone, your skin may require deeper cleansing, particularly of carbon particles. This may sound complicated, but basically you are loosening the particles (including the ones you cannot see) that have adhered to the skin and wiping them away.

HOW TO CLEANSE

1 Moisten a cotton makeup pad with water and use it to wet your skin's surface slightly.

2 Apply a little cleanser to the pad and gently wipe away the surface grime and makeup. Start with the nose, then the forehead, and then the remainder of the face (use more pads and cleanser as necessary). Use a soap-free cleanser around the delicate eye area. Always use a separate pad for blemished areas to prevent the spread of bacteria.

3 Repeat step 2 to cleanse the skin itself.

4 Blot (do not rub) the skin with a facial tissue to remove oil traces.

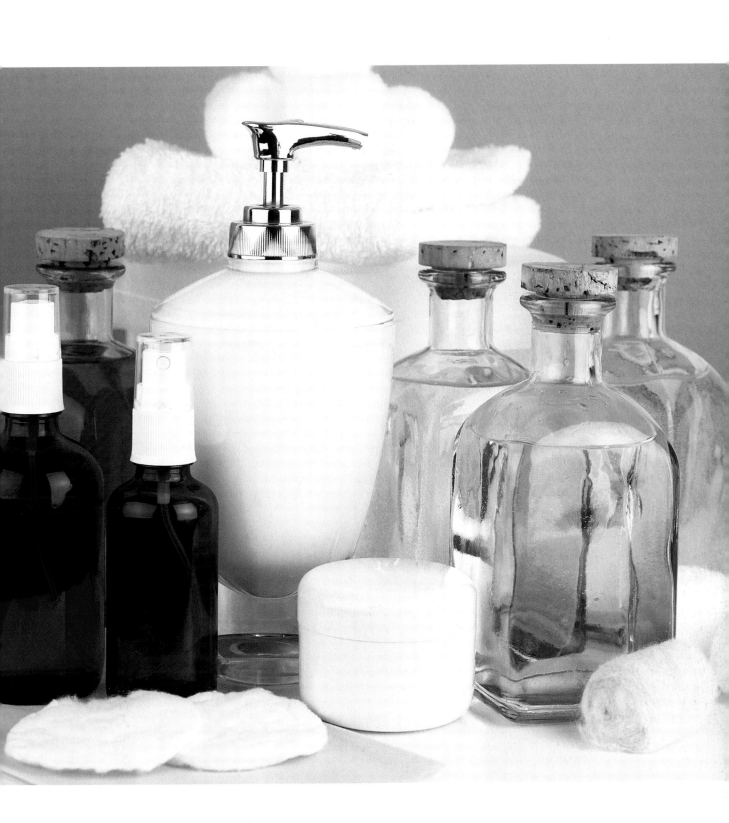

ABOVE *Everything you need for your daily skin-care routine – cleanser, toner, eau naturelle spray, and moisturizer.*

CLEANSING CREAM

This is an oil-based cleanser, although it does not have an oily texture. Add herbal and floral additives to this basic recipe to make this cleanser suitable for your skin type (see chart opposite). You can also use this cleanser as an eye-makeup remover, but you must omit the natural soap.

Makes 2 x 50g jars

INGREDIENTS

PART 1

5 tsp oil, such as almond, apricot, or peach kernel oil
9g emulsifying wax or 10g beeswax

PART 2

70ml purified water or rose, lavender, or tea tree water
1 tsp vegetable glycerin
5 drops lemon juice
1 tsp very finely powdered handmade natural or gentle soap
   (omit if using cleanser around the eye area)
Active ingredients (see chart opposite)

EQUIPMENT

Measuring spoons
Scales
Double boiler
Thermometer
Flameproof jug
Juice squeezer
Stirring spoon
Balloon whisk
Screw-cap jar

PART 1

1 Put the ingredients into the upper pan of the double boiler. Fill the lower pan with hot water. Gently heat until the mixture reaches 150–160°F or the wax has dissolved. This is what is known as making an emulsion. Pour into a jug and set aside.

PART 2

2 Put the ingredients (except the active ingredients) into the upper pan of the double boiler and fill the lower pan with water. Keeping Part 2 on the heat, slowly pour in Part 1, keeping the mixture at 150–160°F and stirring quickly. If the mixture cools, the wax may separate. If this happens, gently reheat and keep stirring until the wax dissolves again. Whisking gently may improve the emulsions.

3 Remove the mixture from the heat and stir until it becomes milky. Keep stirring (or use an electric mixer on low speed), checking that you incorporate all of the mixture at the bottom and sides of the bowl.

4 When the mix starts to thicken and turns white, add any active ingredients (see chart opposite). Stir to blend completely and whisk until the mixture becomes thick. Put your cream into a screw-cap jar and label it. Store in a cool place and use within 6 weeks.

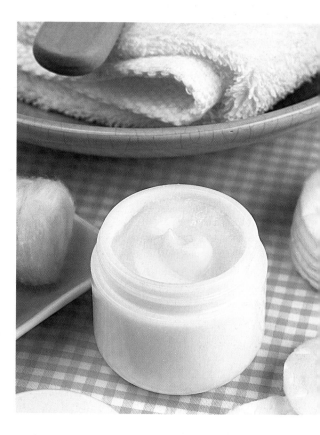

ABOVE *Natural handmade soap grated to a very fine powder may be added to your recipe.*

The glycerin helps remove stubborn makeup and makes the skin feel soft and smooth.

ACTIVE INGREDIENTS These can be added to cleansers, toners, and moisturizers

SKIN TYPE	normal	normal / dry	normal / oil rich	oil rich / combination	blemished / acne
APPLE CIDER VINEGAR (5%)			5ml / 1 tsp per 100g	5ml / 1 tsp per 100g	5ml / 1 tsp per 100g
CALENDULA INFUSED OIL (10%)					10ml / 2 tsp per 100g
CARROT INFUSED OIL (10%)	10ml / 2 tsp per 100g	10ml / 2 tsp per 100g	10ml / 2 tsp per 100g	10ml / 2 tsp per 100g	10ml / 2 tsp per 100g
CEDARWOOD ESSENTIAL OIL (2%)			2–4 drops per 25g	2–4 drops per 25g	
CLARY SAGE ESSENTIAL OIL (2%)			2–4 drops per 25g	2–4 drops per 25g	2–4 drops per 25g
EVENING PRIMROSE OIL (10%)	10ml / 2 tsp per 100g	10ml / 2 tsp per 100g			
FRANKINCENSE ESSENTIAL OIL (2%)	2–4 drops per 25g	2–4 drops per 25g			
GERANIUM ESSENTIAL OIL (2%)			2–4 drops per 25g	2–4 drops per 25g	2–4 drops per 25g
HONEY (5%)			2ml / ½ tsp per 100g	2ml / ½ tsp per 100g	2ml / ½ tsp per 100g
LAVENDER WATER (10%)	Replace half the water in recipe	Replace half the water in recipe	Replace half the water in recipe	Replace half the water in recipe	Replace half the water in recipe
LAVENDER ESSENTIAL OIL (2%)	2–4 drops per 25g	2–4 drops per 25g	2–4 drops per 25g	2–4 drops per 25g	2–4 drops per 25g
ROSE ESSENTIAL OIL (1%)		1–2 drops per 100g	1–2 drops per 100g		
ROSE WATER (10%)	Replace half the water in recipe	Replace half the water in recipe			
TEA TREE ESSENTIAL OIL (2%)				1–2 drops per 25g	1–2 drops per 25g
TEA TREE WATER (10%)			Replace half the water in recipe	Replace half the water in recipe	Replace half the water in recipe
WITCH HAZEL WATER (10%)			Add 5ml / 1 tsp to finished recipe	Add 5ml / 1 tsp to finished recipe	Add 5ml / 1 tsp to finished recipe

* When combining essential oils and botanicals, do not exceed 2% in total of one or a combination of essential oils and a maximum total additives of 10%. Any more may cause separation. Maximum percentage of use in a finished product is shown in brackets.

* When buying and using essential oils, read the instructions carefully because a number of them are not suitable for certain medical conditions, such as pregnancy and high blood pressure.

TONING

A toner is an astringent – it finishes the cleansing process, closes the pores, and reduces the chance of impurities entering the skin's delicate surface. A toner's astringent properties may also help to calm overactive secretions, which can give skin an oily, shiny appearance. Using a toner also removes any remaining cleanser and tap water and helps restore the skin's slightly acidic pH balance (4.5–6).

HOW TO TONE

1 Depending on the kind of container that your toner is in, either spritz the face (keeping the eyes closed) or apply with a cotton pad, avoiding the delicate eye areas.

2 Wipe the toner gently across the face and neck.

SOOTHING TONERS

Here are three different recipes for toners, each one tailored to a specific skin type.

Makes a 50ml bottle

INGREDIENTS

FOR OIL-RICH AND BLEMISHED SKIN

2 tbsp witch hazel water
1 tsp lemon juice
1 tsp apple cider vinegar
40ml purified water

FOR SENSITIVE AND DRY SKIN

50ml rosewater
25ml aloe vera juice
2 drops frankincense essential oil
2 drops sandalwood essential oil

FOR BLEMISHED, PROBLEM SKIN, PRONE TO BREAKOUTS

50ml tea tree water
1 tsp lemon juice
2 tsp witch hazel water
1 tsp apple cider vinegar

EQUIPMENT

Measuring spoons
Measuring jug or beaker
Juice squeezer
Bottle or screw-cap jar

1 Put all of the ingredients into the bottle or jar and secure the lid. Shake well, so that the ingredients mix. Shake well before each use.

Beauty tip

An eau naturelle spray of purified water or water with a 20-percent addition of floral water infusions (see page 83) can give your skin a refreshing lift and freshen your makeup. Use low sodium mineral water and change the water in the bottle daily. A spritz to the décolleté and back of the neck is also refreshing and calming.

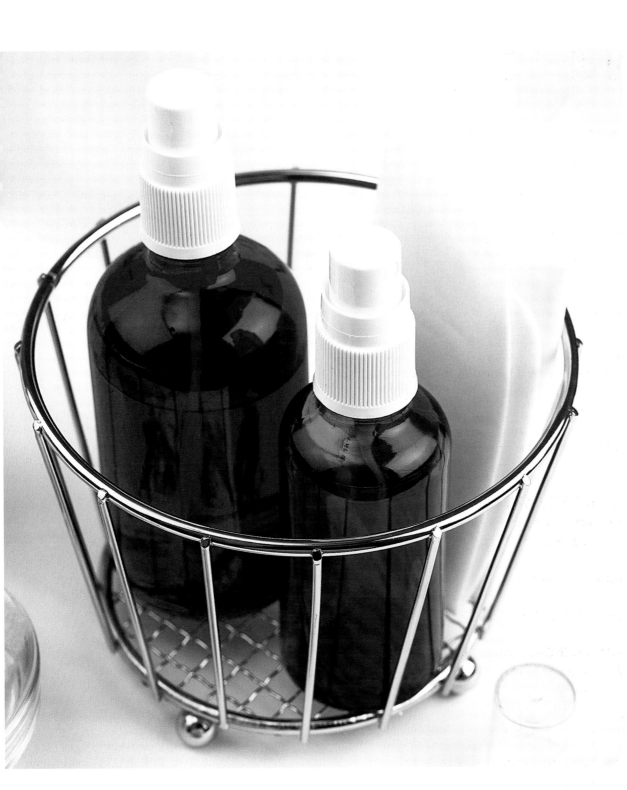

ABOVE *Make a selection of eau naturelle sprays so that you can use them at different times of the day. Sometimes your skin can feel dry and tight in the morning, yet be prone to oiliness in the evening. Work with your skin and respond to its needs, rather than trying to use just one product.*

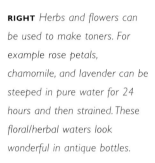

RIGHT *Herbs and flowers can be used to make toners. For example rose petals, chamomile, and lavender can be steeped in pure water for 24 hours and then strained. These floral/herbal waters look wonderful in antique bottles.*

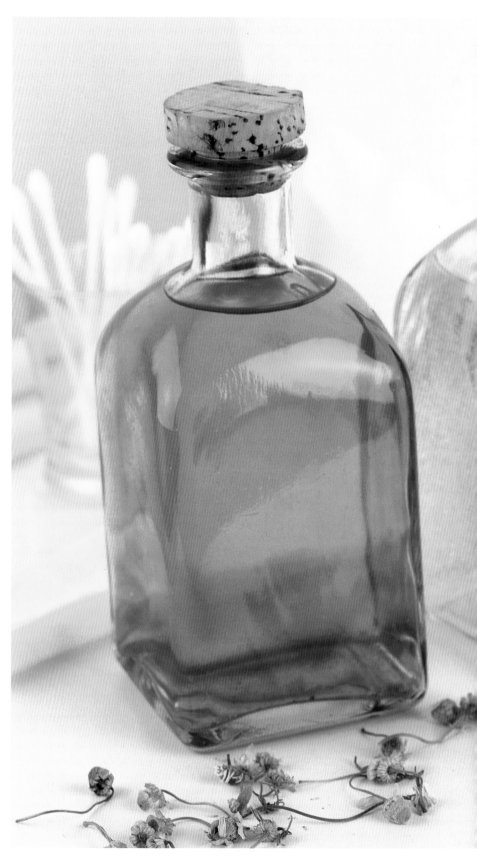

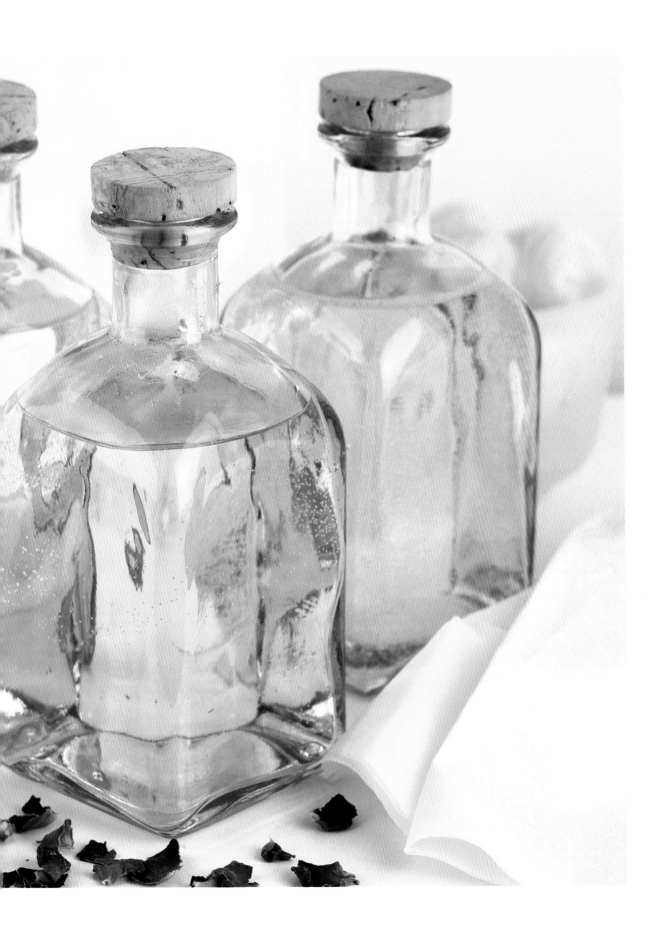

MOISTURIZING

The main purpose of using a moisturizer is to help the skin hold moisture and retain its elasticity. Using moisturizer before the toner dries seals the active ingredients into your skin. Allow at least 30 minutes after applying moisturizer before putting on your makeup. This gives the moisturizer time to rehydrate and revitalize the skin. Adding a drop or two of fresh lemon juice to a moisturizer acts as a natural antiseptic for problem skin and helps the skin maintain the correct acid balance. You can add pigment tints to the moisturizer recipe below. Just follow the color guidelines given for the Foundations (see pages 62–63) and use approximately half of the color pigment additives. Gently whisk into the finished cream, following the rules of color preparation.

HOW TO MOISTURIZE

Moisturizer should be applied gently following the natural contours of the skin and underlying facial structures. It should be applied with a light touch either with the fingertips or a soft foam or cotton pad. Never drag the skin and always allow the moisturizer to "work" before applying foundation. Moisturizer should be reapplied several times a day. I knew a photographic model who applied moisturizer at least 4–6 times a day, and her skin was wonderful. Refresh your supply of moisturizer regularly and always store it in a cool place. It's best to keep it in a pump dispenser as they are hygienic and easy to use.

Apply a generous layer of moisturizer before you go to bed; this allows the skin to absorb the rich natural oils. Cleanse, tone, and moisturize again in the morning.

LIGHT CREAM MOISTURIZER

This light, refreshing cream is suitable for use during the day and won't make your skin feel at all oily. If you wish to make the cream richer, perhaps for use at night, substitute half of the apricot kernel oil with avocado oil. Add additional active ingredients for your skin type.

Makes 2 x 50g jars

INGREDIENTS
PART 1
25ml apricot kernel oil
25ml jojoba oil
10g emulsifying wax or 15g beeswax

PART 2
70ml purified water
2 tbsp rosewater
1 tsp lemon juice
Active ingredients of your choice (see page 83)

EQUIPMENT
Measuring cup
Scales
Double boiler
Heat-resistant jug
Measuring spoons
Stirring spoon
Balloon whisk
Screw-cap jar and label

ABOVE RIGHT *This light moisturizer gently freshens and rehydrates the skin.*

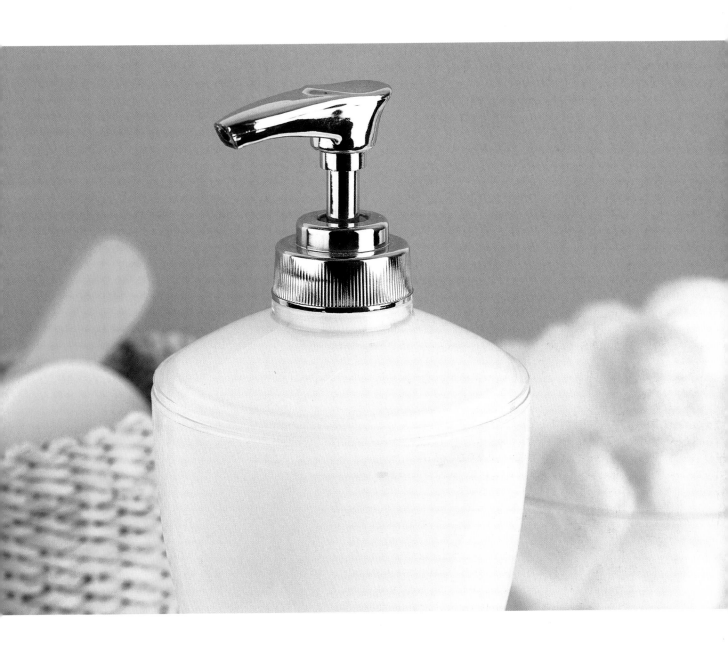

PART 1

1 Put the ingredients in the upper pan of the double boiler. Put hot water in the lower pan. Gently heat until the mixture reaches 150–160°F or the wax has dissolved. Pour into a heat-resistant jug and set aside.

PART 2

2 Put the ingredients (except the active ingredients) in the upper pan of the double boiler. Put water in the lower pan. Gently heat. Keeping Part 2 on the heat, slowly pour in Part 1, keeping the mixture at 150–160°F and stirring quickly. If the mixture cools the wax may separate. If this happens, gently reheat and keep stirring until the wax dissolves again.

3 Remove the mixture from the heat and stir until it becomes milky. Keep stirring (or use an electric mixer on low speed), checking that you incorporate all of the mixture at the bottom and sides of the bowl.

4 When the mix starts to thicken and turns white, add any active ingredients (see page 83). Stir to blend completely and whisk until the mixture becomes thick. Store your cream in a screw-cap jar and label it. Store in a cool place and use within 6 weeks.

TROUBLESHOOTING

There are all sorts of reasons why sometimes things don't quite turn out as you'd hoped – maybe you've used a slightly different product, the conditions in which you prepared the recipes were either very hot or cold – it could be anything. The most important thing is not to be deterred from trying again – your knowledge and skill will improve with experience. Listed below are some of the problems that can occur, along with the reasons why and what you can do.

EYES

Powder eye shadows crumble easily – add 1 or 2 drops of jojoba oil to bind.

Powder eye shadows are sticky – add a little more talcum.

Crème eye shadows are sticky – add a little talcum.

Crème eye shadows are too oily – melt gently and add a little more wax to bind.

Cannot fill straws with mixture for color sticks – reheat the mixture and increase the temperature slightly; the mixture should be thinner and therefore easier to pour.

Color sticks too soft – add a little talc and carnauba wax. You can reheat and improve the recipe if you need to.

Mixture runs over the top of color sticks – simply wipe away the excess to leave a clean, even surface.

Color too strong – soften with talcum and titanium dioxide or use the appropriate colors to subdue the shade. For example, use blues and greens in tones that are too red and add iron oxides to tones that are too blue or green.

Color too pale – carefully blend more pigment.

Color streaks – indicates that pigments were not prepared sufficiently – small lumps and air pockets remain. Wax-based makeup may be re-melted as further stirring may help incorporate the color.

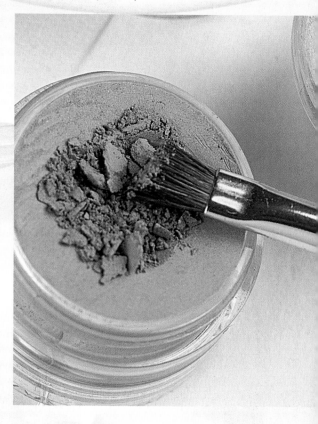

FACE BASE

Foundation gives shiny appearance – add more talcum.

Foundation too matte – add a little more oil and balance with a touch of natural mica.

PARTY TIME

Henna paste not creating enough color – warm the paste, add a little more lemon juice and a few more drops of essential oils, and let it cure for 1–3 more hours. Applying the color when it is warm (you must make sure it is not too hot) is sometimes more beneficial to certain skin types.

SKIN PREPARATION

Creams/emulsions separate – melt half of the quantity of wax listed in recipe (i.e., if original recipe required 10g wax, melt a further 5g). Warm the cream to 98–104°F. Add the melted wax to the warmed cream and whisk. This should stabilize your mixture.

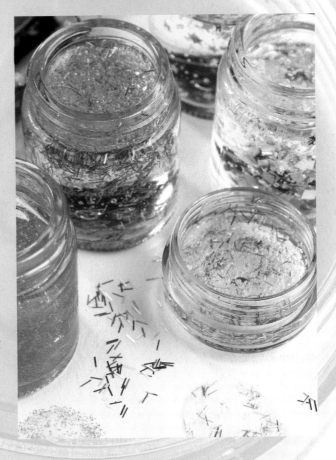

LIPS

Lip colors appear the same in recipes – the subtle differences in color make a great deal of difference in the finished makeup. Follow the recipe; if the color is too pale or too dark, balance with your shades to improve to suit your complexion.

Lipstick from homemade mold needs shaping and looks dull – gently cut and sculpt the tip into a "bullet" point. Dip the tip quickly into boiling water; this will smooth the surface. The same method may be used to polish the surface or you can wipe it with a clean nylon stocking to improve the gloss effect.

GLOSSARY

Absorbancy The ability of a product or your skin to absorb products, moisture, oils, or color.

Acid balance Skin's natural acid mantle or condition.

Additives Ingredients added to a product to preserve, color, texturize, perfume, etc.

Adhesion Ability to remain on the skin for a time.

Antioxidant Product that prevents fats from spoiling and improves the skin, clearing free radicals that cause damage and sensitivities.

Antiseptic Helps to prevent infection from forming and spreading.

Applicator sponge, cotton ball or swab, brush, or fleece for applying makeup.

Astringent Ability to close pores.

Balancing Restoring to equal condition.

Barrier Preventative product to assist the skin in repelling a substance, i.e., color pigments.

Binder Ingredient to help the product remain in a solid, emulsion, or stick form.

Botanicals Plant materials.

Buffer Product to resist change in pH.

Cellular regenerator Assists the skin's natural ability to heal and repair.

Compact (1) Storage container for foundations, powder, and shadows.

Compact (2) Pressure to force particles of a powdered product to fuse and become a solid mass.

Concealer Camouflage agent.

Concentrate In an unfinished form that requires further extension to become a finished item.

Dehydrated Lacking moisture or water.

Dyes Materials that color the product rather than stain the skin.

Emollient Improves elasticity and softness.

Emulsion Oil in water or water in oil blend of products to make a stable mixture.

Emulsify To combine oil and water into a stable solution.

Emulsifier Product with the ability to stabilize and prevent separation of oil and water emulsions.

Essential oil Pure plant extract produced from distilled botanical sources.

Fats Oils and butters such as olive, almond, shea butter, etc.

Fixative Product that helps perfumes and essential oils retain their aroma and active effects.

Fixed oils Vegetable and nut oils (may be termed as fats) that do not evaporate or solidify at room temperature.

Fragrance Perfume components to give aroma to a product.

Formulation Recipe ingredients that will produce a given product.

Glitter Light-refracting sparkle ingredient. May be natural or synthetic.

Godet Shallow metal tray filled with makeup and inserted into decorative compact.

Highlight Give a lightened and lifted (brighter) color effect.

Holographic Multicolored and multifaceted effect produced by microscopic iridescent colored layers.

Infused oils maceration Soaking of plant material in cool, fixed oil for a period of time (usually four weeks) until the active botanical compounds have become "fixed" or suspended in the oils.

Interference color Microscopically layered light-refracting and reflecting particles to give shimmer and sparkle for added interest in a product.

Iridescence Light-reflecting and shine created by additives.

Iron oxide Inorganic compound used to impart color in cosmetics and toiletries.

Mascara tube and wand Cylinder with reducer and brush-tipped applicator, which may vary in size as to its ability to curl, lengthen, and bulk the product on the lashes.

Moisturizing An emollient product to make the skin feel softer, smoother, and more supple.

Mold Form that is filled with raw product which is allowed to set, thus adopting the shape of the mold.

Mortar and pestle Bowl (mortar) and pressure/grinding/pulverizing tool (pestle) set, which has been used to pulverize materials and foodstuffs for thousands of years.

Natural A product created in a living environment and not manufactured in a laboratory.

Ointment An oil mixed with wax to form a solid to enable application.

Opaque Cannot see the underlying form beneath it.

Pearlescent An effect that gives a "color" and appearance of pearl (or mother-of-pearl shell).

Pigments Color materials.

pH Acidity or alkalinity of a product. Normal skin pH is 5.5–6.5.

Preservative Protects products from contamination by micro-organisms. These could be introduced in manufacture, by raw materials, or by the user and storage conditions. The important issue with preservatives is that they protect both the product and user. They often have bad publicity when tests show the raw materials have negative effects, but they are designed for use as a diluted product and are there for protection, making the product safer and more desirable.

Pulverize To break into smaller and finer particles.

Ramekin Small cookware bowl often used for individual desserts and pâtés.

Silicones A brittle element found in sand, clay, granite, and quartz. They are chemically altered to provide a product resistant to water, temperature and chemicals. Also provide insulation and lubrication.

Sheer Color with the ability to show the skin's natural tones even when covered with product.

Stabilizer Ingredient to prevent a formula from spoiling, separating, or damaging a container.

Temporary (Tattoo) Decoration on the skin that will fade or be non-permanent.

Topical (anti-inflammatory) Product applied to the skin (topical) to prevent inflammation.

Ultramarine Color compounds of reds, pinks, blues, greens, and violets.

Wax Solid or semisolid substances of various origins that enhance the appearance of the skin. Are often standardized, for use in the cosmetics industry.

NOTE ON LEGISLATION

Every country has its own legislation and criteria which must be followed in the interests of safety. All cosmetics sold must have labels that comply with the International Nomenclature Cosmetic Ingredient (INCI) listings. This includes color index (CI) numbers. The regulations are designed to protect the public when offering products for sale. The makeup that you make using the recipes in this book is for personal use only, it cannot be sold.

UK/EU – The Department of Trade and Industry (www.dti.gov.uk)

USA – The Food and Drug Administration (www.fda.gov)

Australia/New Zealand – The Australian Society of Cosmetic Chemists (www.ascc.com)

South Africa – South African Bureau of Standards (www.sabs.co.za)

SUPPLIERS

CANADA

Green Cottage Supplies
11253 Regal Drive
Surrey, BC V3V 2S5
Tel: (604) 584-7627 (information line)
Tel: (604) 584-7627 (order line)
www.greencottage.com
Pigments, colors, raw materials.

USA

The Chemistry Store
520 NE 26 Ct
Pompano Beach, FL 33064
Email: sales@chemistrystore.com
www.chemistrystore.com
*Comprehensive range of ingredient supplies and
containers.*

From Nature with Love, LLC
PO Box 201
Hawleyville, CT 06440
Tel: (800) 520-2060
www.fromnaturewithlove.com
*Cosmetic ingredients, equipment, and packaging.
Shop online.*

Green Girl Basics
46 W. Tulane Road
Columbus, OH 43202
Tel: (614) 263-3938
Email: greengirlbasics@aol.com
www.greengirlbasics.com
*Lip balm tubes, containers, packaging, and cosmetic
ingredient supplies.*

Quosmedix
150-Q Executive Drive
Edgewood, NY 11717-8329
Tel: (631) 242-3270
Email: info@quosmedix.com
www.quosmedix.com
Cosmetic containers and applicators. Mail order.

Snowdrift Farm
Snowdrift Farm, Inc.
2750 South 4th Avenue, Suites 107–108
South Tucson, AZ 85713
Tel: (520) 882-7080
www.snowdriftfarm.com
Range of colors, ingredients and containers.

www.makeyourownmakeup.com
*Online suppliers of kits and ingredients to support
this book.*

Note
**Supplier information is current at the time
of publication. We have made every effort to
ensure the accuracy of content of the
publication. We are not responsible for any
human or typographic error.**

INDEX